OXFORD MEDICAL PUBL

Healthy Respect

HEALTHY RESPECT

Ethics in health care

SECOND EDITION

R. S. DOWNIE MA, BPhil, FRSE
Professor of Moral Philosophy,
Glasgow University

and

K. C. CALMAN MD, PhD, FRCP, FRCS, FRSE
Chief Medical Officer, Department of Health, London
Formerly Professor and Dean of Postgraduate Medicine,
Glasgow University

with a contribution from
Ruth A. K. Schröck MA, PhD, SRN, RMN, RNT
Formerly Head of the Department of Health and Nursing,
Queen Margaret College, Edinburgh

Foreword by
Sir Malcolm Macnaughton MD, FRCOG, FRCP, FRSE
Formerly Muirhead Professor of Obstetrics and Gynaecology,
Glasgow University
Formerly President of the Royal College of Obstetricians and Gynaecologists

OXFORD   NEW YORK   TOKYO

OXFORD UNIVERSITY PRESS

1994

Oxford University Press, Walton Street, Oxford OX2 6DP

Oxford   New York   Toronto
Delhi   Bombay   Calcutta   Madras   Karachi
Kuala Lumpur   Singapore   Hong Kong   Tokyo
Nairobi   Dar es Salaam   Cape Town
Melbourne   Auckland   Madrid
and associated companies in
Berlin   Ibadan

Oxford is a trade mark of Oxford University Press

Published in the United States
by Oxford University Press Inc., New York

A catalogue record for this book is available from the British Library

Library of Congress Cataloging in Publication Data
Downie, R. S. (Robert Silcock)
Healthy respect : ethics in health care / R. S. Downie,
K. C. Calman, with a contribution from Ruth A. K. Schröck;
foreword by Sir Malcolm Macnaughton.—2nd ed.
Includes bibliographical references and index.
1. Medical ethics.   I. Calman, Kenneth C. (Kenneth Charles).
II. Schröck, Ruth A. K.   III. Title.
R724.D687   1994   174'.2—dc20   93-39946

ISBN 0 19 262409 1 (Hbk)
ISBN 0 19 262408 3 (Pbk)

Typeset by Advance Typesetting Ltd, Oxfordshire
Printed in Great Britain by
Bookcraft (Bath) Ltd

FOREWORD
by Sir Malcolm Macnaughton
MD, FRCOG, FRCP(Glas.), FRSE

The ethical aspects of medical care have been with us for a long time but the interest in this area has become much more pronounced in recent years and now 'medical ethics' is a popular subject of discussion by people in all walks of life. This, in turn, has made the medical profession itself pay much more attention to the ethical aspects of health care in its widest sense.

The real stimulus to this widespread interest has been the development of new techniques and new forms of management which have addressed such basic subjects as life and death; fertilization of the egg by the sperm in a laboratory; and the experimentation on embryos which has brought into consideration in a very practical sense the questions: 'When does human life actually begin? What moral status should be given to an embryo? What can and cannot or should or should not be done to an embryo? When does personhood occur?' At the other end of the life cycle, developments in artificial respiration have resulted in keeping patients alive who would normally die and have given rise to the question: 'When is a person dead?'

Health care is a bottomless pit as far as financial funding is concerned. In practical terms finance has to be limited so that there are financial restrictions on health care. This results in, for example, a restriction on the number of patients who can have renal dialysis. 'Who then should be given priority for this treatment and what are the ethics of this?' Problems arise in the selection of patients for dialysis. 'What is the balance in the use of resources?'

The medical profession is basically pragmatic as far as health care is concerned. In general, doctors wish to develop new methods for health care that will improve the quality of the lives of the patients that they treat. They sometimes find it difficult to see why restrictions should be put on when the results are so obviously beneficial. 'What then is meant by quality of life?'

There are a variety of ways of looking at medical care; a variety of arguments that can be advanced and other considerations to take into account which health care professionals may not always consider. At the same time the public, politicians, lawyers, theologians, and others may not always be aware of the problems the health care professional has and they also have to remember who is at 'the sharp end' of the decision-making. The health care professionals have a collective responsibility which, so rightly, has been pointed out in this book and this is sometimes not fully appreciated.

Medical students generally, at present, do not spend much time on the ethical aspects of medicine. When they are being taught about such subjects as *in vitro* fertilization, artificial insemination by donor, terminal care, brain death, renal dialysis, and priorities in care, they are involved in learning the various kinds of decision-making but seldom in their course is there a formal teaching of ethics. This book attempts to remedy this deficiency and the authors have tried to put the arguments for and against the various problems and to ask the student to think about these problems. The student is introduced to the philosophical discussion of the 'slippery slope' argument and the argument of consequences and the various philosophical aspects of ethics. This enables the student to obtain a 'new look' at some of the problems and see some of the fallacies of the arguments that are put forward. It would in fact be most valuable for all medical students to have a course in philosophy related to medicine as part of their medical course and this book attempts to fill this gap. It should be essential reading for medical students and, in addition, all those who think they know the answer to the moral problems discussed here should read this book. In addition to medical students and doctors – lawyers, politicians, and theologians and, indeed, anyone in the general public who seeks to have a view on these difficult aspects of medical ethics, and especially those in public life who can exert influence and perhaps even legislate, ought to read this book in order to acquaint themselves with the difficulties. This would enable them to take part in a much more rational discussion of the problems than has been the case so far. This is a most valuable book and I hope it will be widely read.

PREFACE TO THE SECOND EDITION

In presenting the second edition of *Healthy Respect* we should like to comment on a few changes in the context in which health care ethics is being taught. It is pleasing to note that there is an increasing awareness of the need to include some consideration of ethical issues in medical and nursing courses, and we hope that this book will make a contribution to student discussion in such courses. As we stressed in the first edition, this book is the outcome of joint teaching to medical and nursing students by a moral philosopher and an experienced clinician, now turned medical administrator. We hope that this book will show the advantages of co-operation.

In the few years which have elapsed since the first edition there has been an enormous increase in the public perception and understanding of AIDS, partly the result of public health campaigns. At the present time, however, it is not clear to us that AIDS really raises any new ethical issues, as distinct from requiring careful application of the old and familiar principles. For example, the importance of confidentiality has always been known, but the nature of AIDS and the ways in which it spreads have highlighted its importance. Again, the ethical requirement to obtain informed consent for blood tests has long been appreciated, but, in view of the likelihood of HIV infection in blood samples, informed consent becomes a much more emotional issue. Yet no new issues of principle are involved. There is in any case a large literature on all aspects of AIDS, so we shall not discuss it separately.

We have, however, added a chapter on quality issues in health care. The need for this has arisen because of changes in the organization and evaluation of health care. It is one of our assumptions that moral issues are all-pervasive in human activity; we have therefore added a chapter on the moral aspects of this new concern. Public health and health care economics were topics discussed in the first edition, but in view of their increasing importance we have revised and enlarged our discussion.

It will be noted that in the chapter on 'Learning and teaching about moral values' (Chapter 10) we have added an extended discussion on the use of the arts and literature to raise moral questions in health-care courses. It may be objected that the curriculum is already overloaded and that it is unrealistic and perhaps unjustifiable to expect much by the way of expansion in non-specific subjects. Nevertheless, with such a highly selected and motivated population as present-day medical and nursing students a great deal can be achieved by even a moderate degree of encouragement, combined with increased time available for self-education. For example, most medical schools have 'medical groups' attached—interdisciplinary groups which discuss a range of ethical and related issues. There is no reason why there should not also be encouragement for the setting up of groups to discuss plays, poems, and novels which raise issues of interest to all those in health care. We hope that our book will contribute to the creation of an educational environment in which such enterprise may flourish. Education in medicine and nursing has many excellent qualities but it requires completion and expansion into a broader and more humane world-view. The discussion of ethical questions, whether in moral philosophy, case-histories, or literature and the arts, will contribute to this process.

Glasgow   R. S. Downie
London 1993   K. C. Calman

PREFACE TO THE FIRST EDITION

This book is the outcome of our experience of teaching ethics to medical, dental, nursing, and social work students. It is one of our main themes that, despite the proliferation of books on specialized professional ethics, the essential unity of the health care professions must be emphasized. We therefore hope that physiotherapists, dietitians, pharmacists, radiographers, and other health care professionals will also join us in this exploration of the values of health care, and that what we say will encourage patients — who can be any one of us — to take an interest in the value judgements made by those who care for our health.

Part 1 of the book sets out the moral philosophy of our approach to health care, and Part 2 places the moral philosophy in a clinical context and is in a format useful for discussion. We have provided references back to Part 1 when the themes overlap. Our own experience of teaching is contained in the recommendations of Chapter 10.

We should like to stress one feature of this book — we intend it to be usable by medical, nursing, dental, and other health care students and their teachers. During the last five years many excellent books of 'applied moral philosophy' have appeared, but they are very properly written one step back from the day-to-day problems of health care, and to those students and teachers who do not have a natural interest in philosophical questions they can seem remote. Without at all wishing to suggest that these books are written in ivory towers we unashamedly hope that our book will speak of the dust of the arena. This is especially true of

Part 2. It may be that, having come to appreciate the pervasive nature of uncertainty and therefore of value judgements in health care which we try to portray, readers will develop an appetite for moral philosophy.

We gratefully acknowledge the help of several friends. Dr Ruth Schröck has given us essential advice on nursing and moral philosophy. Her great contribution more than merits her name on the title page. Professor Macnaughton has taken time from his busy schedule as President of the Royal College of Obstetricians and Gynaecologists to make comments and write a Foreword. As a member of the Warnock Committee he is well aware of the pitfalls of ethical debate. Some of our ideas on the moral philosophy of health care were first developed in *Caring and Curing* (1980) of which one author was Elizabeth Telfer, and we are most grateful to her for commenting on Part 1 of this book. The handwriting of philosophers is inscrutable and that of doctors is plain bad. We both owe a debt to Mrs Norma Wallace for deciphering the indecipherable with the equanimity of a good GP and the patience of a good philosopher. Finally, we thank the many students whose disagreement or incomprehension has forced us to be a bit clearer. Our sincere hope is that we shall manage to pass on some of the ideas they have given us.

University of Glasgow   R. S. Downie
May 1986   K. C. Calman

CONTENTS

PART 1

INTRODUCTION

In recent years health care professionals, and the public they serve, have become more conscious of the complexity of the moral dilemmas which can be created by caring for other people. There is now growing awareness of the need to identify clearly what these moral problems are, and to arrive at possible solutions for the patients and for the nurses, doctors, or other professionals concerned, while taking into account wider social issues.

Moral concerns, of course, are by no means the prerogative of the health care professions, although the traditional way of talking about 'medical ethics' or 'professional ethics' may have conveyed the mistaken idea that those who care for others have special claims to knowing or deciding what is right and wrong in health and illness. Moreover, by being members of a profession concerned with the well-being of people, doctors in particular, but also nurses and other health care workers, have allowed themselves to be seen as arbiters in public and private moral dilemmas for which they may have no more expertise than any other thoughtful and considerate person. This book aims at raising the awareness of health care professionals of the moral dimensions of their everyday actions and should be seen as a starting point for an enquiry which can be taken as far as the reader wishes.

A serious examination of moral issues in the context of professional health care need not be characterized by daunting and obtuse language. Moral arguments, when plainly and intelligibly expressed, should be perfectly manageable even by those unfamiliar with this kind of discussion. But the endeavour to avoid unnecessarily difficult language does not make this a simple book. The thoughts, concepts, and arguments which are explored in these pages need the reader's serious intellectual application in thinking them through carefully, and in applying them to his or her own working situation. Moral consciousness cannot be taught or passively acquired by reading a suitable text. Its development requires the active participation of the student in the debate. All readers will bring to this debate their own experience of situations in which questions arose that were difficult to answer. Such subjective experiences are both valid and important. One way to be reminded of them is by hearing or reading of a similar event, even when it does not in all details coincide with one's own experience. For this reason, and to allow the reader to become imaginatively as well as intellectually involved, we offer various scenarios and brief examples of real events, although names and places in particular are entirely invented.

The issues raised in this book are equally pertinent and important to all practitioners whatever the road of their professional preparation may be. We therefore use the term 'health care professional' rather than 'doctor' or 'nurse'. Whichever the professional location, be it as nurse, doctor, or dentist, physiotherapist, speech therapist, occupational therapist, dietitian, or social worker, or any other member of the health care team, questions about what is right or wrong cannot be avoided in the day-to-day encounters with patients or clients, with their relatives, friends, and neighbours, and with colleagues. If such questions are ignored, not only will the distress for others be increased, but one's own position may become very precarious indeed.

Investigations of the sort we undertake in this book are often referred to as 'medical ethics', 'nursing ethics', 'professional ethics', or the like. This usage can be misleading, for the term 'ethics' has various meanings and associations.

First, it can refer to that branch of philosophy also called 'moral philosophy'. Thus, philosophers write books with titles like *Methods of Ethics* or *Principia Ethica*, and such books are concerned with the philosophical study of the principles governing man's life in society. Ethics in this sense is a theoretical study of practical morality and its aim is to discover, analyse and relate to each other the fundamental concepts and principles of ordinary practical morality. Our book, especially Part 1, is an essay in moral philosophy or 'ethics' in this first sense. Our overall aim, however, is not just to provide a theoretical *understanding* of ordinary morality, important though that is, but to contribute to the *improvement* of the practice of health care. Marx tells us that philosophers have tried only to understand the world, whereas the point is to change it, and Aristotle tells us, near the beginning of his *Nicomachean Ethics*, that the end of the enquiry is not knowing but doing. Following them, we hope that 'ethics', in the sense of the moral philosophy provided in Part 1, will illuminate our discussion of the practical moral problems in health care which we initiate in Part 2, and perhaps even lead to the improvement of health care.

Part 2 illustrates the second main sense of 'ethics' — ordinary morality as it is found in a professional context. In this book we shall use the words 'morality' and 'moral decision' rather than 'ethics' and 'ethical decision' to refer to the practical problems we all encounter. There are two reasons for adopting this usage. The first is that it brings out the *continuity* between the moral problems of everyday life and those encountered in hospitals or other spheres of professional practice. We try to emphasize this continuity in Part 2 and in our examples. The second is that the term 'ethics' encourages a narrow view of morality as consisting simply of the 'do's' and 'don'ts' in a code. In our view morality must be seen *broadly* as including the whole area of value judgements about good and harm.

The third sense of 'ethics' refers to codes of procedure, or ethics *narrowly* conceived. These are important for they give some of the principles which underlie professional activity and they apply across cultural and national boundaries. We include some codes of ethics of various branches of health care in Chapter 19 in order to display the consensus which does exist at the level of basic principle. Clearly, however, basic principles cannot encompass the range of moral problems facing health care professionals.

It is worthwhile stressing the difference between the second broad sense of ethics as value judgement which will concern us for most of Part 2, and the narrow sense which refers simply to the items on a traditional list, to be discussed in Chapter 19. For example, in the wide sense it is a moral or value judgement that a given patient, all factors considered, *ought to be allowed* home despite the risk of a recurrence of his problem. But clearly, this decision does not raise a question of morality or ethics narrowly conceived. It is because many health care professions take ethics or morality in the narrow sense that they are unaware of the extent to which they are continually making moral or value judgements in the broad sense. There are certainly technical — scientific and social — factors involved in deciding whether or not a given patient ought to be allowed home. But the decision about what ought in the end to be done goes beyond the technical and encompasses the professional's overall judgement as to what is for the total good of the patient. This overall (all things considered) judgement of the patient's good is what we mean by a moral or a value judgement. One of our central aims is to make the professional aware of the all-pervasive nature of such value judgements and the extent to which the professional's own values affect his decisions.

To sum up, we can say that our book involves 'ethics' in all three senses: as moral philosophy, as moral or value judgements broadly conceived, and as codes or morality narrowly conceived. But since the term is used in these three different senses (at least), and additionally suggests that health care ethics is somehow divorced from ordinary morality, we shall try to avoid the word where possible.

Ideally, a reader should become familiar with the material in Part 1 before discussing the clinical cases in Part 2, but it would be possible in a brief course to take relevant chapters in Part 2 and refer to Part 1. We have provided cross-references.

OBJECTIVES

Our book is directed towards the following objectives. We aim to:

(1) help the student or practitioner of any health care profession, or the general reader, to analyse competently a professional situation or problem;

(2) enable such a person to identify moral issues inherent in professional situations;

(3) introduce a range of moral concepts used frequently in the discussions of professional ethics and to relate them to everyday notions of morality;

(4) encourage the reader to examine his or her own values, beliefs, and attitudes and to relate them to those of others;

(5) enable the reader to give his own views, based on a reasoned and justifiable argument, on a moral issue related to professional practice;

(6) enable the reader to recognize systems of value and views of human nature other than those typically associated with health care.

Chapter 1

KNOWLEDGE, SKILLS, AND VALUES

1. QUESTIONS

This chapter will be concerned with showing how knowledge, skills, and values (both personal and professional) are all involved in health care. As a way of bringing this out by an example and introducing the reader to some of the central concepts, assumptions, and more detailed objectives of the work consider the first of our scenarios.

The accident and emergency department was more than usually busy. Even Sister Maxwell who had seen some hectic days was heard to be muttering,

'This is incredible!'

She grabbed a bundle of dressing pads and rushed down the corridor where she almost collided with Staff Nurse Hanson.

'Where have you been? It really is too much! If you can't be on time, don't bother coming at all!'

Nurse Hanson knew she was about 10 minutes late and generally respected Sister Maxwell for being organized and fair in her dealings with people. But today she felt she had had about enough before even starting. She was not habitually unpunctual and felt quite angry to be received in this way. As she turned towards the office, Dr Sinclair emerged, stopped, and asked,

'What is the matter? You look terrible.'

It was not just the encounter with Sister. She had recently decided, after much worry, to ask her mother to look after her four-year-old rather than pay for a trained child-minder, and now she wasn't sure whether she had made the right decision. This morning she had rushed her child to her mother only to find great confusion there. She now felt guilty about the resentment which came through in her outburst,

'You do pick your time to have one of your ghastly migraines!'

It had not been right for her to say that but she still felt aggrieved. Everybody seemed concerned about patients and mothers and children . . . did they respect her needs at all?

Although she was a good deal calmer by the time Sister returned, it did not help her feelings of injustice to hear Sister greet Mr Smith most pleasantly when he sauntered in about an hour later for the follow-up examination of the boy they had seen yesterday with a pretty nasty cut across his leg caused by his clambering over barbed wire. He was to have been seen at 9 a.m. and now had been waiting for about an hour along with one or two other patients. Did it not matter if consultants were late? She must have been thinking aloud,

'Is there no justice in this world?'

Mrs Miller, the senior radiographer, startled her by saying behind her back,

'What kind of a question is that?'

It is certainly not the kind of question generally asked and far less answered in professional training. Let us therefore begin by looking at the kinds of question which are typically asked and answered on health care courses from medicine and nursing through to social work. In other words, let us look at the knowledge-base of such courses.

Each one within the broad range of the health care professions will have its own particular knowledge-base, although there will be a large amount of overlap. For example, whereas a medical student requires a fairly comprehensive and general knowledge of anatomy and physiology, a speech therapist or a dentist needs a far more detailed knowledge of the anatomy and physiology of the mouth and related areas. It would also be prudent for all health care workers to acquire some knowledge of the law to the extent that it bears on their professional work. We shall later (Chapter 2) examine more theoretically the nature of the professional knowledge-base, but at the moment let us just note that it seems to consist of factual knowledge. This philosophers have sometimes called *knowledge that* certain things are the case. In clinical terms examples of knowledge *that* certain things are the case would include such pieces of information as:

The blood is pumped by the heart to the arteries, the arterioles, the capillaries and returns in the venous system to be oxygenated in the lungs.

The abducens nerve controls the motor function of the lateral rectus muscle of the eye.

Cimetidine is an H_2 receptor antagonist and reduces gastric acid secretion.

These are simple clinical facts known to the appropriate workers. Yet in a historical sense it is important to note that such information was not always available and that in the future new answers and facts will inevitably come to light which may change our whole concept of a particular disease or illness.

It is important to recognize that changing the factual knowledge may change the kinds of decision that have to be made. Take the introduction of cimetidine, for example. Prior to this the management of chronic duodenal ulceration was by simple symptomatic measures such as bed rest or antacids, or by a surgical procedure. The decision as to when to operate was a difficult one. The introduction of cimetidine as an effective non-operative technique for controlling the disease changed the balance of decisions, and introduced a wider choice for the patient and the doctor.

Since all health care professions are practical, their primary aim is doing rather than knowing. But practical skills or *knowledge how* require a factual or knowledge-base, and that is why *knowledge that* is essential for the development of practical skills, or *knowledge how*. Arising from a broad factual knowledge-base there will be a huge range of professional skills, from knowing how to move an overweight patient, how to bypass coronary arteries, to knowing how to interview prospective parents for an adoption. In addition to the practical skills originating in their factual knowledge-bases all health care professions require skills in communicating effectively with their patients or clients. Most training programmes now include some study of and practice in communications.

Like factual knowledge, practical skills are constantly changing and improving. One has only to look at recent developments in health care, transplantation, *in vitro* fertilization, coronary artery bypass procedures, bone marrow transplantation, vaccination against hepatitis, to see how these practical skills may change our views on moral issues, and challenge our traditional values. New procedures and skills will continually evolve and the doctor, nurse, or other health care professional must begin to consider the moral dimension of changing methods of diagnosis, prevention, screening, and treatment.

The process of turning the factual knowledge-base of health care into practical skills is a problem for teachers and students, and we have all experienced how in general such teaching and learning might proceed. But where in all this do we look for the answers to moral questions of the sort which arose for Nurse Hanson, and are they relevant to health care? Is there a special skill in acting justly or in answering moral questions, and if so, can it be learned or taught? How does it relate to the more familiar kinds of *knowledge that* and *knowledge how* to be found in professional training courses?

These questions are very old. They were discussed for example in Plato's *Republic* in the fourth century BC. Plato pointed out that we know what a good carpenter is good at, what his skill is, but what is the good or just man good at? The answer which emerges in Plato's discussion is that there is no specific, separable skill which constitutes being just or being a morally good person; rather, being just or good or compassionate involves qualities which pervade everything one does. It might be helpful at this stage to put it this way: we have already spoken of *knowledge that* and *knowledge how*, and we now suggest that moral knowledge can be seen as at least analogous to that sort of *knowledge by acquaintance* which is knowing a friend. If you know a person well, you don't just know lists of facts about him, or you do not just know how to get him to do what you want or how to cheer him up (although you will also know these things). The point about a friend or someone you love is that you have a certain sort of *attitude* towards him or her; you appreciate and respond to the kind of person he or she is, and you are committed to them. Morality is like this; it is a pervasive concern, affects all our activities and carries commitment with it.

This type of knowledge is based not just on factual information and practical skills, but also on a series of intangibles such as feelings, beliefs, and attitudes. Moral knowledge is influenced by our upbringing, culture, personality, and peer group pressures. Moral knowledge, in this sense, is personal knowledge associated with our own beliefs and attitudes. The point we want to stress by comparing moral knowledge with the attitudinal aspects of knowledge by acquaintance is that it is misleading to think that there are clinical discussions or professional decisions and occasionally also separate moral decisions. Rather, our argument will be that *all* clinical or professional decisions have a moral dimension to them, for morality, like attitudes, is all-pervasive. Moreover, since morality is all-pervasive it cannot be compartmentalized and it is therefore impossible to separate the moral decisions of someone in a professional capacity or role from the moral decisions of that same individual in a private capacity. We tried to bring this out in our example of Nurse Hanson.

We have mentioned the importance for health care workers of developing effective communication skills, but the decision as to *how* and *what* to communicate is a moral matter. Certainly, there is much to be learned from the social sciences about the *how* or the skill of communication. But communication skills ungoverned by moral attitudes become crude manipulation. What is needed in communication skills is not just technique but a humane practice. Indeed, even uneducated patients or clients can sense the difference between tact, charm, or sympathy which are simply 'turned on' as a matter of technique and those which spring from a genuinely caring attitude.

Turning now to the question of *what* to communicate, we wish to emphasize that it is the individual professional's *interpretation* of the available information which determines what is said to the patient or client. In making this point we are challenging the assumption that factual information in some scientifically compelling form is the only determinant of what to communicate.

In most common medical or nursing problems the information available is not always 'firm', and judgement in choosing the appropriate course of action is almost always required. Hence the importance of the moral dimension in clinical decision-making as to what to communicate.

At this point two comments might be made in considering that there is a moral dimension in all clinical decisions. Both concede the importance of moral considerations in professional judgement. First, it could be said that the moral dimension is taken care of by requiring the student to learn the relevant code of ethics of the profession, and second, that the moral dimension is taken care of, not by learning, but by intuition, or, as some would have it, it is just a matter of 'common sense'. The second point might also be put by saying that since moral decisions are based on personal factors no guide-lines could be drawn up to assist *all* health care professionals. Further, it implies that morality cannot be learned.

In replying to the first point we do not deny the importance of codes of ethics to a profession, for we discuss them in Part 2, but these are necessarily limited in scope, consisting only of broad principles which on occasion may even conflict with one another. Moreover, no set of principles can by itself tell us how and when to apply them in everyday life. Further, codes of ethics deal only with the profession's values, not with the patient's values, or the changing values of the wider society in which health care is practised.

In replying to the second point we can again agree with the importance of developing intuitive judgements in morality, as indeed in professional matters generally. The intuitions of an experienced practitioner in his or her field of work are likely to be better than those of an inexperienced person. But such intuitions, whether based on experience or not, may later need to be justified by appropriate observations and debate.

Consider a typical ward round discussion of whether or not a 76-year-old man should be allowed home after a two-month admission because of a cerebrovascular accident which gave him temporary loss of function of the right arm and leg. After considerable rehabilitation it is now time to consider whether or not he should go home. Factual information will be available from tests and from the occupational therapist, physiotherapist, and social worker. Nursing and medical background will also be available. It is at this stage that the personal intuition of all will be brought into play. The question of who should make the decision, and on what grounds, will be left till later in our discussion.

In discussing the importance of 'intuitions' or 'hunches' in clinical decisions it is important to remember that just as our factual knowledge and skills require to be constantly upgraded, so the germs of social feeling which we may be born with require to be developed by use, and extended by reason, and even our mature moral judgements require to be justified to others by argument; 'common sense' is not enough. Our aim is to assist in this process of moral development and the justification of intuitions.

The question of *how* our moral intuitions or perceptions are to be justified requires us to introduce another aspect of the matter − that of logical analysis and argument. So far we have been concerned with the close link between professional knowledge and skills and moral perceptions and have maintained that this link must be defensible. But how? The answer is that the process of justification requires logical analysis and argument. Those whose training has been basically scientific are well aware of the importance of cogent logical arguments in their scientific work, but perhaps less aware that logic can also extend to the justification of moral decisions. We therefore regard it as important to devote some space to logical questions. We do not want our readers to become logicians, but we need to develop a heightened awareness of logical analysis and some of its pitfalls.

Moral judgements, we said, are essentially part of our professional judgements. However, there is also the economic aspect of the matter which is important, but generally ignored in books on professional ethics. In stressing this we are not just contemplating the importance of discussing the comparative cost of various treatments, or the efficiency of a national health service compared with other systems of health care. These are valid questions, but the fundamental point is that all of us engage in economic activity in our daily lives. To do so is to evaluate and choose in the use or the distribution of scarce resources over competing demands. For example, if we should like to spend two weeks abroad for our holidays and also to buy a new car, but cannot afford to do both, then we are faced with the need for a judgement of economic value. We must decide on the relative importance of each alternative in our overall objectives. This example may also serve to bring out the close link between economic and moral considerations.

Almost all health care workers are familiar with the invidious decisions that have to be made where irreconcilable demands are made on scarce resources. For example, both the geriatric unit and the out-patient department are in need of additional nursing help but only one part-time staff nurse is available. Let us assume that both areas have put forward a well-substantiated request and the available staff nurse could help effectively in either situation. What possible criteria or values could influence the nursing manager's decision? Once again a range of factors might be considered, and it is not difficult to see that the economics of health care will affect the morality of decision-making and vice versa. We discuss some practical problems of the economics of health care in Part 2.

So far in this chapter we have considered three types of knowledge which are important in making clinical decisions:

Knowledge that – factual information

Knowledge how – practical skills

Knowledge by acquaintance – the moral dimension of attitudes and value judgements. It has been noted that the moral dimension is important in all forms of decision-making, and that practice is required to improve all three forms of knowledge.

2. ASSUMPTIONS

We are now in a position to make explicit the assumptions on which our book is written. The first assumption is that *morality is inescapable.* In both the domestic and the professional life of our Nurse Hanson, and in the interaction between those aspects of her life, moral considerations arose. The point is that living together with other people requires that we acknowledge certain actions to be right or just or compassionate, and others to be wrong or unjust or inconsiderate. Without some agreement on what we ought to do, and what we must not do, there could be no social harmony and co-operation. What this agreement or moral consensus is we discover in the process of growing up, from the way in which we may praised for doing some things and punished for doing others. In so far as we try to improve the quality of our own lives, and at least in our professional work the lives of other people, we must share some values to determine which direction to take. It may be only at times when what we think is right is considered to be wrong by other people, or when we find it difficult to decide what it is right to do, that we become conscious of a moral conflict. Much of the time when there is no overt disagreement we may not be conscious of the moral nature of our actions precisely because morality is an inescapable part of our lives.

Second, we are assuming that *morality is all-pervasive.* The discussion of 'professional ethics' has tended to highlight the dramatic issues which happen to be topical at any one time. Although euthanasia, abortion, resuscitation, surrogate motherhood, or embryo experimentation are undoubtedly important matters, their prominence has obscured the fact that not just once but many times in the course of a working day moral stances and decisions will result in actions considered to be right or wrong by the professional worker. Whether we value honesty in our dealing with patients more than avoiding the truth (to save time or to avoid disagreement with colleagues or having to justify ourselves) is a matter of morality. Whether we do a job only moderately well when we are capable of doing it better, is a question of morality, of deciding which direction we want to take. Allowing ourselves to become professionally socialized into routine working patterns which keep things going but diminish patients' dignity and freedom requires as much a moral justification, if it can be found, as a sociological explanation.

We assume, third, that *morality is indivisible*. There is a traditional distinction between 'professional ethics' and 'private morality', and to those who draw it the notion that one can deal with moral questions in a professional context without examining personal values and convictions is perhaps not unreasonable. But this is not an assumption on which this book is based. On the contrary, it follows from the inescapable and all-pervasive nature of morality that we encounter moral problems in our personal lives which are not fundamentally different from those we may have to explore in our working environment. We tried to bring this out in the episode of Nurse Hanson. Whatever values we may feel to be important to us as individuals are almost certainly influencing and directing the decisions that we make as professional health care workers. If we have or lack the skills which allow us to approach moral dilemmas in a rational and methodical way, this will affect how we attempt to solve moral problems in a professional context.

On the other hand, this fundamental assumption about the 'indivisibility' of morality does not lead to a rejection of the very special place that the maintenance of acceptable professional standards of behaviour must have in the work of people whose primary responsibility is to care for vulnerable fellow men and women. The potential harm that can come to people who are in some ways and by definition dependent on the knowledge and skills of others will undoubtedly heighten the moral concern in situations which, outside the professional context, might not be perceived as quite so threatening or acute. For example, a critical or sarcastic remark, which might be acceptable in ordinary circumstances, could be devastating to a sick person.

Another aspect of our 'indivisibility' assumption is that hospitals and other health care organizations are not immune to general attitudinal changes in society. Moral dilemmas arise frequently from the attempts which the professions make or do not make to accommodate social change. Likewise, what professional people do, or often more pertinently what they would refuse to do, reflect the moral standards of their society in the same way in which the actions of the individual doctor or nurse, psychologist or speech therapist, social worker, or dietitian reflect his or her standards of personal morality.

A fourth assumption is that *moral decisions must be made in the real world of scientific and economic facts*. Some people conduct moral discussions in terms of absolutes. From one side we hear that there is an absolute value on human life, that abortion, or euthanasia, or experiments on embryos are always wrong; while another side insists that a woman has an absolute right to choose on matters such as abortion, that patients' rights always take precedence over any other consideration, that parental rights are paramount, and that informed consent must be given for every medical intervention. We hear from others that conventional, mechanistic, hospital-based medicine is always inferior to holistic medicine or herbal cures, or that testing on animals is always wrong. No doubt a debating case can be made out for all such positions, but our view is that in the real world compromises must be made. As an example of compromise we can point to renal dialysis. It is not helpful to say that there is an absolute value on human life if there are two patients who would benefit from dialysis but facilities for treating only one. Again, it is irresponsible to say that abortion is always wrong when you will be driving some desperate women to a back-street abortionist or even to suicide. Again, it is wrong to wage a one-sided campaign against the use of animals in medical experiments while there are still millions of animals needlessly suffering for the purposes of the cosmetic or other luxury trades.

Our view is that there are two sets of information which while they do not determine nevertheless set the scene for any moral judgement in health care: the indications of a well-substantiated professional assessment, and the economic resources available. It is in the light of these that most moral decisions on health care must be made. We recognize this, and therefore express our fourth assumption in the form of a distinction between compromising our consciences, which is wrong, and conscientious compromises, which consist in making the moral best of a bad job in the light of the two sets of facts we have noted. Our fourth assumption is compatible with the view that in some circumstances no compromises should be made.

Our fifth assumption is that while the morally good person has neither a special sort of knowledge nor exactly a special sort of skill, *morality is learnable and teachable*, up to a point at least. Obviously, the non-moral basis of moral decision-making is learnable and teachable. As we have seen, this consists in the factual knowledge and practical skills, including communication skills, of the health care professions. These are a central concern of professional training, and we shall say nothing about them, except to stress their importance from the moral point of view. Moral decisions are what can be called 'consequential' or 'resultant' in that they arise out of the professional, economic, and legal facts of given cases; ethics is no substitute for a good diagnosis of the problem or skilfully carried out treatment or clearly communicated information.

Another aspect of the non-moral basis of moral decision-making consists of the agent's ability to conduct a logical analysis of a situation. This involves skill in handling conceptual frameworks, awareness of what constitutes a better or worse argument for an adopted position, and the imagination to enter into points of view other than our own. We hope that our whole book will help with the learning and teaching of this, and in particular we have included a special section on common types of logical argument in moral contexts to assist both students and teachers.

This same learnable logical skill can also raise awareness of the subtle ways in which the academic disciplines which contribute to the knowledge-bases in the preparation of the professional worker may influence the perception of what might be justifiable behaviour in a professional relationship. Most of these disciplines in the health care field are, as we have seen, of a scientific and practical kind, bringing with them quite specific assumptions about the nature of human beings, the possibilities and potentials of human life, the proper solutions to human problems, and even the nature of human society.*

*See Chapter 7, section 2; Chapter 8, section 1.

Turning now to the central question of whether morality itself can be learned and taught, we hope that the main contribution that this book offers to the student as well as to the practitioner of any of the health care professions is an example of how moral philosophy (or the study of ethics) can find a valid and relevant place in their professional studies. Since teaching and learning about morality, about what is right and wrong in personal or professional terms, is not like studying those disciplines which are more familiar to the health care professions, this book will not be like any other textbook. Morality is not a matter of instruction but a matter of judgement. Therefore this book cannot satisfy those who seek an 'instruction manual' to the proper conduct expected of them; yet it might help those who are willing to be guided to find their own solutions to the moral dilemmas in their professional work. In Chapter 10 we offer some detailed suggestions on learning and teaching which may be useful.

It must be stressed that our five assumptions simply give a general idea of our approach. They are neither necessary nor sufficient to characterize the nature of morality, a question which in itself needs further exploration (Chapters 3–7).

3. CONCLUSION

1. Morality is inescapable, it is part of life.
2. Morality is all-pervasive, it is not just a matter of the 'big' issues, but is associated with all our clinical decisions.
3. Morality is indivisible, it cannot be divided into 'professional' ethics and 'private' morality.
4. Moral decisions must be made in a real world, in which changing clinical practice is constantly challenging our moral attitudes and assumptions.
5. Morality can be learned and can be taught. As a corollary to this there is the assumption that moral values can change, and that it is possible to look at the reasons behind the moral values we hold.

The main components contributing to a justifiable moral decision and consequent action in a professional context can be shown as follows:

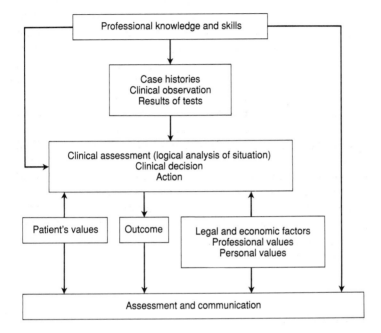

Chapter 2

SCIENTIFIC UNDERSTANDING AND DECISION-MAKING

Moral problems involving the caring professions are generally newsworthy. For example, the Warnock Committee Report on surrogate motherhood and experiments on human embryos has received a large amount of publicity. Issues of death and dying, of consent to treatment, of private medicine, or of the influence of the drug industry on health care are never long out of the news. Debates of this sort are healthy and to be encouraged, but they have one drawback − they can suggest that moral problems are always dramatic, episodic, and carry specific names, whether well-known ones like euthanasia and abortion, or the new abbreviations such as AID or AIDS. These issues all give rise to important moral problems, but as we argued in Chapter 1, moral problems and value judgements are much more pervasive than debates on the headline-catching issues might suggest. Indeed, our main theme was that almost all of the decisions we make in relation to patients have a moral dimension. An examination of decision-making in the caring professions will develop this point more clearly.

1. THE TECHNICAL MODEL OF DECISION-MAKING

The health care professions are pre-eminently practical in that they are concerned not simply with adding generally to our knowledge or skills, but with carrying out a variety of specific actions and policies aimed at effective health care. Moreover, they act in relation to *individual* patients or clients or to *specific* communities. It follows from this that the basic question of any health care worker is: 'What ought I to do for the best care of this patient, or this community?' In other words, the fundamental question of all caring is individualized, and has an 'ought' in it. It is not asking: 'What in general *is* the case?' A question of the latter sort is a scientist's question and is answered by the provision of scientific knowledge, whereas the basic question of care is practical and cannot be answered only by information as to what is the case. To answer a practical 'ought' question is to make a *decision* about what ought to be done.

However, there are close links between scientific questions about what is the case and practical questions about what ought to be done. Consider the following example. A young person goes to his general practitioner with a bad skin rash. The general practitioner obtains some information about the patient's age, diet, and occupation, and prescribes a certain ointment. The elements of this situation are (1) that the patient wants to be cured, (2) that the general practitioner wants to help his patient, and (3) that he has some relevant scientific knowledge and experience of similar problems. In other words, from the facts that someone wants something, that a practitioner is willing to help, and that there are particular means to achieve what the patient wants, it seems to follow that a specific decision ought to be taken.

This example seems to illustrate that while health problems are indeed practical, to be resolved by decisions about what ought to be done, the decision itself is based on scientific knowledge and experience. The 'ought' is there all right, but it is a scientific or technical 'ought' rather than a moral one.

This is a plausible analysis, and it can be applied to many practical situations. For example, let us imagine someone who wants to buy a house, or who wants a divorce, and goes to a solicitor. The solicitor will decide in the light of the client's wants and his own knowledge of the law what ought to be done. Thus we have another professional context in which there are: (1) desires for a given objective; and (2) knowledge of the best available means. Together these entail an 'ought' which resolves the practical problem, but, as in the previous case, the 'ought' is a technical one, and once again there seems no moral element. This technical model of decision-making is persuasive and deeply-rooted in the health care professions. It flourishes especially at this historical period when all the health care professions are striving to become more technical and to build up their expertise. Unfortunately, it is not only an over-simplified model but it is also misleading. It conceals from health care practitioners and the general public the pervasive nature of moral and value judgements inevitably made in the diagnosis and treatment of patients or clients, and indeed in the assessment of the success or failure of such treatments. It is therefore important to bring out where the technical model is deficient, and this is our main justification for spending some time on the nature of scientific understanding. Having discussed the salient features of science and social science we shall proceed to stress the uncertainties and evaluations involved in applying science and social science to health care, and the consequent evaluative nature of the decisions finally reached. We hope that we shall thereby be able to suggest a more satisfactory model for decision-making in health care.

2. SCIENTIFIC UNDERSTANDING

Historically speaking there are few natural sciences which have not been thought relevant to health care, and especially to medicine and nursing. Apart from the biological sciences, which have always been considered to be pertinent, medical practitioners in ancient times looked to astronomy for assistance and now turn, in a variety of ways, to mathematics, physics, and computing. It would seem, then, that there is no one type of science which is uniquely relevant to medicine, and indeed what is called 'medical science' is just a convenient label for a group of sciences studied by medical students; what is included in this group will vary to some extent from one historical period to the next. It might therefore be helpful to enquire whether there are any characteristics shared by all the sciences. Is there something we could call 'the scientific approach to the world' which would be the real basis of medicine and nursing and indeed of other health care practices? What are the main aims of science, and how do scientists proceed?

The *first characteristic of scientific procedures* we shall note is that all sciences, whether physical, biological or social, are concerned with the search for patterns or uniformities in their subject matters to explain observable phenomena. Obviously, orders of many varieties can be traced in nature, from the microscopic to the macroscopic. From another point of view we could say that nature can be looked at in different ways according to the purposes of the scientists. Let us look at examples of these orders.

The most basic of these types of uniformity, the concern of non-numerical science, involves the *uniform association of properties*, such as 'iron rusts in damp conditions' or 'common salt dissolves in water'. The perception of uniformities of this sort is important for the classification of things into kinds. For instance, chemical substances can be distinguished by us because we find that certain attributes of matter uniformly carry with them certain other attributes, and biological species can be distinguished because we find that there are uniform associations of attributes in living organisms. The perception of uniformities of this sort is really just a systematic extension of the discrimination of the world into 'things'. Thus, there is no sharp line between our common-sense knowledge of the world in terms of its 'things' and scientific knowledge. The basis on which the medical scientist begins his investigations is the series of classifications we call biology, and biology is simply the drawing of attention in a systematic way to the properties possessed by different types of living things.

In a clinical sense, this approach is best seen by the way in which we classify disease, its causes or its treatments. Thus illnesses may result from structural damage caused by trauma, by infectious agents, bacteria or viruses, or by degenerative processes. Such a classification allows for the grouping of disease. In a more detailed way it is possible to classify bacterial organisms into different groups – staphylococci, streptococci, bacilli, etc. This approach helps not only in identification but provides information on the nature of the illness, and the type of treatment which might be used.

Thus the search for patterns can provide valuable information which can then be used for the development of practical skills to deal with the problem. In this sense the scientist is analogous to the physician who is charting the patterns of health and illness.

Moving from the classifications of biology to other types of order or uniformity with which scientists are also concerned, we find scientific laws dealing with the *uniformities of change or development* to be found in natural processes. Laws of this kind are common in biological sciences; they might state the stages, say, in the development of an embryo, or in the course of a disease. For example, it is a law of the development of an embryo that the formation of the lungs never precedes the formation of the circulatory system.

Other examples would include the ability to predict the pattern of illness, its symptoms or possible response to treatment. This is often known as the natural history of illness and provides the health care professional with knowledge of what normally happens in particular circumstances. For example, a sore throat and cough are generally related to a simple bacterial or viral infection which should improve spontaneously in a matter of days. If it does not, then a persistent cough or sore throat falls outside the 'natural history' of a simple condition and therefore requires investigation.

Let us turn now to *quantitative laws*. First, there are quantitative laws dealing with numerical *constants in nature* such as the tensile strength of bone or skin. Another type of quantitative law deals with *functional relationships* between measurable quantities, such as the law that for any gas $PV = KT$ (where P stands for pressure, V for volume, T for absolute temperature, while K is a constant depending only on the units of measurement chosen). The functional relationship need not be simple but may be of any type recognized in mathematics. The example of blood flow through arteries falls into this category.

Quantitative laws of the last two types have been formulated only in the more recent stages of scientific development, and sometimes they can be regarded as refinements of previously known qualitative laws. For example, it was known in prehistoric times that iron melted at a great heat, and a quantitative law expressing on a scale of temperature precisely at what point iron melts can be regarded as a more precise formulation of this early perception. Again, it was known from early times that a projectile follows a curved path, but Galileo was able to show that the path is a semi-parabola. More recently a third sort of quantitative law has become important: a *statistical* law. Laws of this kind are to be found in physics, in biology and also in the social sciences.

The importance of quantitative precision in science is so great that some scientists argue that no law is properly scientific unless it is purely quantitative. The arguments behind this view are that true science must be precise, and only the quantitative is precise; that true science must be beyond the subjective or the realm of personal opinions and interpretations, and only the quantitative takes us beyond this realm. These arguments are not convincing. First, laws such as the developmental ones earlier mentioned do not seem to be open to quantitative formulation, but they are still precise. Second, even quantitative laws are concerned in the end with *things* of certain kinds and so they can never be assimilated entirely to purely mathematical formulae. Third, some laws, such as the statistical ones we mentioned, are quantitative but cannot be absolutely precise since they express only probabilities. Fourth, even the quantitative can be open to different interpretations, as is notorious in the case of statistical findings; it is naïve to think that only the qualitative is controversial.

A *second characteristic of the procedures of science* is the use of hypotheses. A hypothesis is a postulated explanation of an occurrence, or of a law. Moreover, it is a postulation from which implications may be drawn which are capable of experimental test. For example, the incidence of a high level of dental caries in a given area might be explained on the hypothesis that the water was too soft. This hypothesis would yield the possibility of experimental testing. If the water were proved not to be soft then the hypothesis would be disconfirmed. If the water were proved to be soft then there would be some probability in the hypothesis, but many more tests would be needed, and even then the hypothesis would be no more than probable because another hypothesis, that too much sugar was consumed, might also explain the phenomenon.

We can generalize the logic of hypotheses in science as follows. A scientist may know that if hypothesis H is valid, then consequences p, q, r must follow. He may be able to devise experiments to check whether these consequences do follow. If they do not follow then H can be rejected. But if p, q, r do follow, then, whereas they render H more probable, they do not logically establish it, because it may be that H2 could equally explain the occurrence of p, q, r. Moreover, even if experiments *disconfirm* a hypothesis, the disproof is conclusive only against a background of assumptions which are not themselves questioned in the experiments. Thus, the logic of hypothesis testing may be set out as follows. Let us call the assumptions K.

1. If H(K), then p, q, r . . .

   But p, q, r . . . are found not to be the case. Then most likely H is false, but perhaps K is false or both are false.

2. If H(K), then p, q, r . . .

   But p, q, r . . . are confirmed, then H(K) is probable, although H2(K) may also be probable.

We can draw some important conclusions from this account of hypotheses. The first is the tentative nature of scientific findings, always open to revision in whole or in part; the second is the close connection between hypothesis and experiment in science; the third is the importance for the scientist of being aware of the background assumptions (K) he may be making. We shall illustrate the clinical use of hypotheses in Part 2.

We have been arguing that science helps decision-making first by establishing patterns and laws in nature which are an important part of the knowledge-base of health care, and second by formulating hypotheses which can yield explanations and further possibilities of observation and experiment. But there is a *third characteristic of science* which can help in decision-making. This is by the development of models, or paradigms, for the way in which nature operates. We are especially concerned with the use of models for the way in which the body and mind function in health and disease.

In breast cancer, for example, the model, or paradigm, which was used to treat the disease some years ago was that the disease began in the breast then spread outward. Using this model it was clear that the most appropriate treatment was to carry out as radical an operation as possible to remove the disease as it spread outward. But experience began to suggest that this method of treatment did not change the natural history of the disease and therefore another model or paradigm had to be developed. Such models, common to all the health care professions, must regularly be challenged, not only by reviewing the available evidence but also be seeing the evidence from different angles.

The philosopher Ludwig Wittgenstein speaks of a fly in a bottle trying to escape. It repeatedly buzzes against the same point in the glass, when all it needs to do to escape is to change direction, for there is no stopper in the bottle. Similarly, the solution to an intellectual or practical problems may be obtained by looking at it from a fresh angle, or by changing the questions one is asking.

To sum up so far this account of the natural sciences, on which so much health care expertise is based, we can say that they give us understanding of the world by using observation and experience to trace various patterns or uniformities, some quantitative and some qualitative, and that they explain the world to us (1) by showing how the events in which we are interested can be fitted into these patterns; (2) by developing hypotheses to predict the future course of events; and (3) by using models to provide a manageable way of looking at a complex set of events.

3. SOCIAL SCIENCES

Carrying this analysis of the natural sciences over to social sciences we can say that social sciences will attempt to trace the patterns or systems which shape human wants and objectives.

Some of these patterns are economic, some political, some legal, some religious or ideological, some psychological. Knowledge of these patterns is undoubtedly of great assistance in understanding human behaviour in general terms. Like the natural sciences the social sciences also use hypotheses and models, such as 'rational economic man'.

In tracing the patterns into which human behaviour tends to fall, social scientists frequently use the term 'social role'. While there is no unambiguous use of the concept, far less a single definition of it, it is a useful tool of social science in that it can act as a bridge concept to explain the influence of society on the conduct of the individual. Thus, individuals act in society *as* labourers, builders, musicians, farmers, teachers, doctors, probation officers, or fathers, where these terms indicate a social function. A nurse, for example, may occupy several roles – a nurse, a wife, a mother, a citizen. While individuals act in these roles, thus contributing to the maintenance of society, the roles in turn shape and influence the whole personality of the persons who act in them. We shall discuss further and make use of the concept of a role in Chapter 6.

A knowledge of the social sciences is essential for any adequate understanding of individual action, because the influence of society is present in every individual action. This point, which has long been recognized in the education of the social worker, has come to be appreciated by the other caring professions. Thus, it is accepted that social influences affect the course and incidence of disease, and also people's toleration of it. Indeed, the very recognition of a state as being 'illness' can be affected by social factors.

4. APPLYING SCIENCE TO DECISION-MAKING

In order to bring out the complexity involved in applying the systematic information of science and social science to the actual decisions of what ought to be done in specific cases let us return to Nurse Hanson, Mr Smith, and his young patient with the nasty cut across his leg caused by his clambering over barbed wire.

Mr Smith's initial good humour had evaporated somewhat when he saw Jimmy's leg from which Nurse Hanson had carefully removed the bandage. It should have been a fairly straightforward matter now, after the wound had been sutured very competently by the accident and emergency SHO on Jimmy's arrival yesterday, when he had also given the lad the necessary anti-tetanus injection.

But how did he get himself and his dressing in such a filthy state in less than 24 hours? The risk of infection with these ragged wound edges was high and by the general drift of the somewhat limited conversation with Jimmy's older sister who had come with him, Mr Smith was by no means convinced that the usual procedure of leaving the wound uncovered and prescribing an antibiotic spray would work.

But he really could not admit an otherwise perfectly healthy boy into the already over-stretched surgical ward with his waiting list growing by the minute. Neither was there any point in asking the health centre to find a district nurse to take on this case. They were struggling to cover far more urgent situations. If Jimmy were to be admitted, he would have to stay the week until the sutures could be removed, otherwise there was no point in keeping him at all. But in a week . . . Mr Smith sighed with exasperation . . . how could one weigh the possibility of a very bad wound infection in a young boy against the certainty that two middle-aged men could get their hernias repaired?

There is no doubt that Mr Smith is struggling with a practical dilemma: he is not sure what he ought to do, what the best means of doing it might be, and whether he will succeed in any case whatever he decides to do. When he thinks about the problem he will clearly be assisted by his knowledge of science, social science, and economics, but these disciplines cannot completely determine his decision about what he ought to do. Let us consider why.

There is a science of bacteriology and a great deal is known about the circumstances in which in general a wound becomes infected. But Mr Smith is not sure whether in this case it will; his information is incomplete and not entirely certain. This is typical of clinical situations even when they do not have the other complexities of our example. The uncertainty and incompleteness of the evidence mean that a decision even on the purely scientific aspects of a clinical problem must be tentative, like the propounding of a hypothesis to be tested by further observation.

In clinical practice such hypotheses are frequently raised and tested, even in very straightforward situations. For example, the laboratory results suggest that a bacterial culture from a patient would be sensitive to a particular antibiotic. By prescribing this antibiotic the hypothesis is tested.

This also implies that in some circumstances the information is not complete and that clinical decisions cannot be determined only by the weight of the evidence; a value judgement is required. To take our example further, suppose the bacterial culture showed that the organism was sensitive to two antibiotics, of which one was cheap but known to have a 5 per cent risk of side-effects, and the other was twice the price but had a 2 per cent incidence of side-effects. How should the doctor choose?

It also emphasizes that decision-making is associated with probabilities. This is best illustrated by considering the difficult question of prognosis. Take a patient with advanced ovarian cancer, in which the recorded prognosis (taken from observation and a review of the literature) is that the patient will, on average, survive nine months. This is a probability which must be translated into the particular, and communicated to the patient. The difficulties with this are apparent and will be discussed later, but highlight the problems of translating factual information into clinical decisions.

In the technical model of decision-making there are three elements: it is assumed:

(1) that the patient or client wants to be helped or treated;
(2) that the health care professional wants to give this help;
(3) that the health care professional knows the best available means to provide this help.

Putting these three elements together we obtain the technical decision. The practitioner ought to do X. We have tried to bring out the complexities in the third step. Even if a practitioner has a good knowledge of the relevant sciences he will still be faced with uncertainties in deciding on the 'best available means' in a given situation. Uncertainties mean choices and, as we shall see, value judgements.

5. APPLYING SOCIAL SCIENCE TO DECISION-MAKING

Let us now turn to the uncertainties of applying social science to Mr Smith's case and other health care situations. We shall be concentrating here on elements (1) and (2) in the technical model − the patient's and the health care professional's wants − although we have already seen in the problems of the comparative costs of antibiotics that economics is involved in the choice of the best available means.

Mr Smith has drawn inferences about Jimmy's social background from the conversation with Jimmy's sister, and he hazards a guess as to the degree of priority which the case would be given by a health centre or district nurse. He also weighs the economic factors − keeping a young boy in the surgical ward for a week against repairing the hernias of two middle-aged men and the appropriateness of antibiotics at widely differing price ranges which we have already mentioned. Now undoubtedly knowledge of psychology, sociology, and economics are all relevant in helping Mr Smith to reach his decision but, as with the scientific factors so it is with the social sciences, incomplete information and uncertainty lead to the forming of tentative hypotheses. We shall try to explain why this must always be so when the social sciences are applied to particular cases in health care.

The social sciences, as we said, investigate the complex factors of social class, status, sex, fashion, economics, and many others which may influence the patterns of human behaviour both for individuals and for communities. Knowledge of those social sciences is clearly important for any health care practitioner. But when they are applied to given individual cases limitations arise which throw the practitioner back on his own judgements.

The first limitation is that human beings are motivated by so many different factors whereas the social sciences, by their very nature as sciences, must deal with abstracted models, with, say, 'rational economic man'. Second, people put different weight on these factors. For example, the views of a patient on a particular course of treatment might vary, depending on the weight the patient puts on such social factors as distance from the hospital, family circumstances or employment. Studies of the 'role of the patient', however helpful, still fall short of enabling us to be sure that we understand what it is for *this* specific individual to be a patient; a given patient may not follow the standard pattern or role. These two points may be combined if we stress that it is an essential feature of human beings that they can exercise *choice*. Choices may or may not follow standard patterns or roles, they may or may not be informed or rational, and even when they are both informed and rational they may reflect a different set of values from those of health care advisers. This means that there will inevitably be uncertainty in the interpretation of the wants of the consumers of health care and a consequent uncertainty in the wants of the practitioners. Let us try to illustrate these points.

In the case of Mr Smith and his patient the boy may well have his own preferences about how he wishes to be treated but the example assumes that the boy has a straightforward desire to have his leg mended in the most efficient possible way, and the uncertainties are seen to be on the part of Mr Smith — elements 2 and 3 in the technical model. Sometimes, however, the uncertainties arise over element 1 — the patient's wants.

First, patients may be confused about their wants. For example, a patient may present with one problem — a skin rash, perhaps — but may really want to talk about some other problem — maybe that he is not happy at home. Alternatively, the patient may not always fully realize that this is what he wants to talk about. Social workers must be familiar with this sort of situation. Similarly, a patient in hospital may request a nurse to help with some need or discomfort, but really wants company for a few minutes. Second, the simple model of decision-making presupposes that there is only one thing a person wants, whereas he may have several, sometimes incompatible, objectives. For instance, someone may want to pursue his ambition in a successful but stressful career involving much travelling, elaborate meals and highly pressured work, while at the same time he may also want to lose weight and lead a close family life. Third, the model presupposes that no one else's wants may be involved. But sometimes it may be in the interests of and indeed be the desire of one person to retire early to escape from a stressful occupation, or a polluted working environment, whereas it may be in the interests of his dependants that his full salary continues to be available.

Moving from element 1 in the technical decision model (the patient's or client's wants or choices) to element 2 (the professional's wants and choices) we can note, fourth, that while the professional by definition concerns himself with the health of his patients or clients, he will be aware that time spent with one patient or client may be at the expense of time or institutional accommodation available to other patients or clients. We have seen that this was one of Mr Smith's problems. He may also consider that some of his time is needed for research for the benefit of many people, or for the wants of his own family and friends. Similarly, at the level of health economics, care is a scarce and expensive resource, and if there is to be more money, say, for renal dialysis, which some patients want, there may be less for the care of children or the elderly, which is what others want. The original model of decision-making must therefore be amended to incorporate the complexities of the wants and choices of patients, clients, and also of professionals.

The professional's decision on all these uncertainties — whether the uncertainties of the diagnosis and prognosis or the uncertainties of the choices and objectives — are made in a social context. The practitioner will be influenced in his decisions, first, by his awareness of the professional opinions of his colleagues on cases of the kind with which he is dealing. Second, for some cases at least he may be aware of the state of public opinion, or legal opinion. For example, the treatment given to neonates with Down's syndrome reflects not only the practitioner's own views but is bound to reflect also those of the parents, his professional peers, the law, and public opinion.

Clearly, then, all three elements in the technical model of decision-making have considerably more complexity than first emerged, and moreover they are made in a complex social context. Let us sum up the information available to Mr Smith or any health care practitioner when faced with a difficult decision.

A good and well-informed practitioner can obtain help from the following sources:

1. Basic sciences, which provide knowledge of the pattern of change and development of injuries, diseases, and all natural and pathological states.
2. Social sciences, including economics, sociology, and psychology, which provide knowledge of the patterns of human behaviour.
3. Collective professional opinion on cases of certain broad types.
4. Legal opinion.
5. Public opinion.

In the light of the understanding which comes from all those sources of information a decision must be made. But how? Are the uncertainties to be resolved by quite arbitrary decision? The answer is that a good health care practitioner will have another sort of understanding of the individual case in addition to that provided by the natural and social sciences. This second sort of understanding involves awareness of moral values, and we shall now turn to an initial analysis of it.

6. TWO KINDS OF UNDERSTANDING

Scientific understanding, as we have described it, is a matter of fitting events into a pattern, of tracing systematic connections. Moreover, scientific understanding is concerned with things in their generality, with the common or universal properties of things or events, or with models. And the same is true of the understanding which the social sciences give of action. They are concerned with what a typical patient or disturbed adolescent might do, or they are concerned with 'people in stress situations', or the 'one-parent family'. Understanding of this kind, however important, is not the same as the sort involved when we suddenly see, or slowly come to realize, what it is for a specific, named individual, now standing in front of us, to be a patient, or to be in a specific situation of stress. Understanding of the latter sort is concerned with actions in their *particularity*, with the uniqueness of situations. We might put the point differently by saying that whereas science, including the social sciences, gives us *horizontal* understanding we must in concrete situations supplement this by what we could call *vertical* understanding, the sort of understanding which comes from insight into a personal history.

Moreover, the second type of understanding of human beings, as distinct from the scientific sort, necessarily requires that one has developed in oneself a certain range of moral qualities, and especially compassion. What these are in detail and how they can be developed we shall describe in later chapters (see especially pp. 51−62). But at the moment our assertion is that we cannot properly understand other persons unless we see them as having various wants and values of their own, and calling forth our respect for that reason. The point here is not yet about how we ought to *treat* another person but is rather the prior point that an adequate *understanding* of another person requires a moral maturity.

This claim can be supported in various ways. For example, it is a moral criticism of someone to say, 'He doesn't understand me', for it suggests that the person is lacking in some sort of moral vision and is seeing one's doings in a cynical or biased way. Of course, there are templates of cynicism which one can impose on the world, just as there are religious and ideological templates. Our claim is that these templates, in terms of which one understands other people, reflect one's own moral values. Sometimes the German word *verstehen* is used to express this concept. It literally means 'understanding', but of the kind we aim at when we try to put ourselves on the inside of the actions of others and capture their meaning for them. Interaction theory sometimes uses the expression *empathy* in attempting to describe the process of understanding an action from the inside. But however we describe this kind of understanding, it is essential to complement scientific understanding and social science understanding in the attempt to reach a humane and appropriate decision.

The decision reached in a health care situation, then, ought to reflect the understanding which a good practitioner has gained from science and social science. But such understanding will still leave uncertainties in the face of the complexities of actual situations. These uncertainties will be resolved by the good practitioner by the exercise of a second sort of understanding, which is perfectly familiar to us since it is the sort of understanding which a friend shows to a friend. It is the sort of understanding which comes from an imaginative and sympathetic insight into a specific situation, and it reflects our awareness of moral values.

7. CONCLUSION

The aim of this chapter has been to show that moral values are inextricably bound up with decisions in health care about what ought to be done. It is not that there are technical problems and separate moral problems; the two are united in the understanding the professional has of patients or clients and in the choices which are the outcome of that understanding. We tried to bring this out by setting up a simple, technical model of decision-making:

1. Patient A wants objective B (cure, treatment, advice . . .)
2. Professional C also wants objective B (to help his patient . . .)
3. Professional C, as a result of his training in science and social science, knows D which are the best available means to bring about objective B
4. Therefore, professional C ought to prescribe or recommend D.

This technical model of decision-making can be criticized on two main grounds:

(a) Elements 1–3 are much more complex in real cases than they seem to a detached theorist. As a result, the sort of understanding which comes from science and social science leaves uncertainties and cannot fully determine the decision.

(b) There is a second sort of understanding, not recognized in the technical model, which is of the first importance in health care. This second sort of understanding is a kind of sympathetic and imaginative awareness of what it is like to be a patient or client in a given situation, and it involves the exercise of moral values.

As a postscript to this chapter we must try to prevent two misunderstandings. We are not saying that in every health care situation practitioners are agonized in their scientific and moral judgements. In many cases the diagnosis and prognosis will be clear and the moral judgement unnoticed because it is uncontroversial. For example, if a woman arrives in hospital to have her baby and the pregnancy has been straightforward then the decisions are not difficult, for the scientific and moral judgements involved will be widely shared by all members of a caring community. Nevertheless, the decisions are still a fusion of the technical and the moral.

Second, we are not saying that it is only via decisions that morality enters health care. Morality may enter health and welfare in a variety of ways. For example, at any given historical period there will be political or community values concerned with health care; again, a profession will have its own values and, given individual practitioners, will *carry out* their decisions and treatment in more or less humane and imaginative ways. For example, a woman having a baby may find it more or less easy to have a place in an appropriate hospital or to have her baby at home – these problems reflect political or community moral values; she may find her practitioners more or less sympathetic to her desire to have her baby at home or in some other manner of her choice – these problems reflect professional values; and she may find in pre-natal and ante-natal care, and in the actual labour itself, that midwives and doctors are more or less understanding of her individual needs – this reflects what we shall later call the morality of role-enactment. We shall come to all these other aspects of the morality of health care in Chapter 6. But our next task is to give an account of moral values, and in particular of the moral values underlying health care.

Chapter 3
MORAL VALUES

Any attempt to give an account of the moral values underlying health care practices is immediately beset by a number of difficulties. Some people say that what is important is the law; that the law creates rights and lays down the obligations of professional practice, and defines such concepts as 'informed consent'. Others say that science, especially the behavioural sciences, can determine moral values, in the sense of showing us how they are really just preferences which can be quantified. An older view, but still widespread, is that it is religion that really determines moral values. Perhaps the most common view among young people is that the whole idea of moral rules is misleading. In the end, according to this view, what people hold to be right or wrong is just a matter of opinion, of subjective taste; there is no possibility of rational argument since your moral decisions are 'just what you think'. All such views are exaggerated or distorted versions of partial truths and we shall begin by showing what truth is in them. The conclusion which will emerge is that while some values change and many factors influence them there is a widespread consensus on moral values which is the foundation for evaluations in health care.

1. LAW AND MORALITY

As far as the law is concerned there must clearly be a close connection with morality since they have concepts in common such as justice, rights, rules, responsibility, and many others. We shall shortly see why this is so, but note to begin with that, historically speaking, each has influenced the other. For example, the development of humanitarian movements in the nineteenth century was influential in the reform of the law on a range of criminal and civil issues. Equally, the change in the law affecting homosexual practices following the Wolfenden Report has had the effect of making people generally more tolerant towards homosexuals.

Despite these historical influences, however, the relevant point for our purposes is that the law and morality are *logically* distinct. A law is legally binding if, and only if, it is recognized by the courts according to the agreed legislative procedures of a given legal system. Legal justice, rights, and responsibility are all equally definable according to the procedural rules of the legal system. The questions of what, morally speaking, the law *ought* to be, of who *ought* to have legal rights and what their content *ought* to be, or of what the criterion for responsibility *ought* to be, are not answered by the law.

To sum up, morality remains undetermined by law and can act as a critique of the law. The connection between law and morality is that what people consider to be of basic moral importance to their lives − their physical and mental well-being, the stability of their property, their liberty, their equality before the law − are matters which the law enshrines and protects with its sanctions. That is why they have concepts in common. It is therefore possible to discover a lot about prevailing morality by analysing current laws, but law and morality remain distinct and independently definable.

2. SCIENCE AND MORALITY

It is not plausible to say that science *determines* morality, although scientists are able to throw a great deal of light on various aspects of morality. For example, neurologists are able to correlate certain areas of the brain with conscience, or a sense of moral right and wrong. But this no more shows that brain activity determines right or wrong than the fact that areas of the brain are correlated with reading or spelling suggests that the meaning of words is determined by brain activity.

Social scientists, again, can correlate different moral attitudes with different sorts of upbringing and different home environments. But this does not mean that our conscience or our moral values are 'nothing but' the voice of our parents. Some philosophers refer here to what they call the 'genetic fallacy' – the confusion ('fallacy' is perhaps the wrong word) between an account of the causal origins of something, of the conditions in which it tends to develop, and of its justification (see p. 126). Even if we suppose that it is true that our moral judgement on something is influenced by what our parents said or did, this fact on its own does not make the judgement morally acceptable or unacceptable – it all depends on what our parents did say!

It is the task of psychologists, sociologists, and other social scientists to *describe* what is the case, what people in fact do, and perhaps neurologists can correlate moral judgements with brain activity. But it is a different kind of task to *evaluate* moral judgements and help the moral agent to decide what he ought to do, and the aim of this book is to show how the moral philosopher might help with this. These points are sometimes summarized in the slogan that you cannot derive a moral 'ought' from an 'is'.

3. RELIGION AND MORALITY

For many people religion is an important determinant of morality. But yet it is entirely possible to maintain the independence and autonomy of morality without attacking religion, and many devout believers do concede the independent existence of morality while retaining their faith. There are several different ways of looking at the connections between morality and religion in the Judaeo-Christian traditions without disturbing the independence of either.

The first of these connections is the *historical* one. It is the case that many of the moral attitudes and practices in Western civilization are directly influenced by Judaeo-Christian traditions, just as they have been influenced by legal traditions. But this is no way shows that morality *logically* depends on religion for its validity. It may well be that without this religious tradition certain moral values would not have emerged, but now that they have done so they can, as it were, stand on their own two feet and be accepted as valid independently of their religious associations. For example, it is possible to accept as a moral principle 'love your neighbour' without being committed to any formal religious beliefs. Indeed, the original explanation of who one's neighbour is — in the parable of the Good Samaritan — makes the point that a person does not need to share one's religious beliefs (if any) or one's race to be one's 'neighbour'. In other words, it is a sufficient reason for helping another human being that that person needs one's help. It would seem then that there is support in the New Testament itself for the view that people in need make moral claims on us independently of any religious framework.

A second connection between morality and religion is in terms of the *practice* of the moral life. Some religious believers feel that they receive help in the difficulties of leading a good life through prayer, divine grace, or religious rules of life. For such people their beliefs are a comfort and an inspiration. But it does not follow from this that those without such beliefs cannot have other resources to help them lead a good life. For some people it is their family and friends who inspire them, for others it is a teacher, for others it is a more abstract ideal or cause. The point is that there can be motivation of various kinds, and whereas religious belief may be necessary for some people to encourage and lead them on their pilgrimage, it is not necessary for all, for there can be other inspirations to lead people in the practice of the moral life.

A third possible connection is probably the most important for it attempts to tie morality essentially, by its very nature, to religion. We shall call this the *essential connection* view. There can be various forms of it and we shall look briefly at two of these. The first is that what makes actions right or wrong is the fact that God has commanded or forbidden them. He creates rightness by his command. It will be apparent why this sort of view is appropriately called an *essential* connection view. The difficulty with it is that if it is taken strictly it makes morality entirely arbitrary. Rightness is thought to be created by arbitrary command, as a tyrant might decide on laws by whim. If it is said that this could not happen because God is good and righteous, then of course we must be assuming that goodness and rightness are not created by command, and the thesis contradicts itself.

The second version of this view is much more appealing. It is that *in* leading a morally good life one is, by that very fact, fulfilling the plans and purposes of God. As the poet George Herbert puts it in his poem 'The Elixir':

> Who sweeps a room as for Thy laws
> Makes that and th' action fine.

The point here is not that we cannot lead a morally good life without religious belief but rather that seeing the duties of ordinary life, however drab, as part of God's purposes gives them a significance that otherwise they might lack. For many health care workers and patients this will be a way in which they can see their lives as meaningful. Their faith will be that the boring duties of life and its suffering are part of a larger plan, and if they could only understand the total picture it would make sense. This kind of faith can also be important in sustaining people in the anxieties and ultimate sadness of terminal care.

But no matter how appealing such a faith may be there is nothing in the logic of morality that obliges one to accept it. There are other possible views of the world as well as the religious one and therefore other ways of seeing morality as meaningful. Whether, then, we think of the historical influence of religious ideas on morality, or the way in which religious belief can affect the moral practice of an individual, or the possibility of a religious framework giving meaning to life, we are not in logic compelled to accept that there is an essential connection between morality and religion; other influences, inspirations and frames of reference also operate.

Moreover, while a religious background might give a basis for making moral decisions it may not be sufficient to deal with new moral situations. This will require a *personal* interpretation of a biblical statement to meet the individual circumstances. The fact that Christians may be divided on their views on abortion is an example of this. Again, the whole enterprise of artificial reproduction raises moral issues, as we shall see (Chapters 5, 13), which cannot be settled by appealing to what God has ordained, for no one knows what has been ordained on such a specific topic.

4. SUBJECTIVE TASTE AND MORALITY

This view, stated in general terms, is that moral beliefs and practices are endlessly varied and therefore there is no one phenomenon which can be identified as 'morality'. Hence, there is no real subject matter for moral philosophy, as distinct from the sociological or psychological charting of beliefs and practices and their correlation with more general personal and environmental circumstances. This objection can be called the moral 'fragmentation thesis', but before we consider it let us dispose of one possible source of confusion.

Our philosophical search for the fundamentals of morality is a search for *principles*, for beliefs about how people morally *ought* to behave. It is not a valid objection to this endeavour to say that people do not always *in fact* behave as they *ought*. Our concern is with principles not with practice, except to the extent that observed practice is a guide to principles which people may hold.

Turning now to the fragmentation thesis we agree that morality is not a monolithic organization of global dimensions. Clearly, it exhibits diversity of various kinds, and the analysis in this book will be concerned mainly with the morality of Western civilization and will not pretend to cover the various moralities of other civilizations, although in Chapter 8 we shall make an attempt to discuss some other outlooks. Indeed, even within Western civilization, there are different ideologies, including liberal-democracy, communism, and various forms of the Judaeo-Christian religious traditions. But the force of this fragmentation or relativistic argument is often exaggerated, for three points can be made to qualify its force.

The first is that despite the undoubted differences which are to be found in the moral principles of persons or communities influenced by the various ideologies of Western civilization, there still remains an underlying similarity in the basic operative principles. This is evidenced in the fact that their representatives (and those of other ideological groups) were able to sign the United Nations Declaration of Human Rights. Certainly, there were important differences in the interpretation of the Declaration, but the fact that it was signed indicates that in very general terms there was a consensus on the broad principles of social morality. In other words, we are claiming that there is sufficient structural similarity in the social moralities of the various communities in Western civilization for present purposes; for we are concerned with the elucidation of concepts and broad principles of morality rather than with local, racial, or class variation of detail in codes of individual morality.

The second point which can be made in mitigation of the fragmentation thesis will be developed in more detail in the next section. At the moment, however, we shall simply state it in general terms. If social morality, whatever else it is, is at least a system of social organization which enables human beings to survive in communal living, then all continuing social moralities *must* have certain structural features in common. They 'must' otherwise they will collapse through internal discord and strife.

Third, let us suppose that no single real-life system of social morality exhibits in its purity all the features which we shall attribute to 'morality'. Let us say for the sake of argument that contemporary social morality in the West is composed of an inconsistent mixture of liberal principles such as Kant's 'respect for persons' principle, of traditional Christian teaching, of the residue of courtly traditions of chivalry, and of folk traditions of morality more ancient and primitive than any of these. It would follow that any attempt to build up a picture of morality in terms confined, say, to the liberal tradition must be subject to the important qualification that no actual moral or political system would conform exactly to such a description. But it would not follow that a picture of social morality created in terms of predominantly liberal ideas would have no theoretical value, for it is by means of such an idealized picture that we may hope to understand something of the rambling structures which are our actual moral and political systems. To understand the complexity of real-life systems we often need the aid of a simple model; this is as true in moral philosophy as in science (see pp. 28–9). Models are representations of a real or actual object and enable us to communicate ideas and concepts. Hence, even if the maximum force is conceded to the objection that social moralities vary from one community to another, or even within the same community, it would not follow that the enterprise of clarifying morality was misguided.

5. CONSENSUS PRINCIPLES

Let us assume as a starting point that, whatever else morality may be, it is at least a set of principles which helps us to live together in society more harmoniously and co-operatively than we could without it. Morality may also have a spiritual dimension, as we have allowed, but it is at the least a social device. If we now consider certain obvious facts about human beings and their situation in the world, we can understand how it comes to be that people have an interest in accepting certain principles of behaviour.

For example, human beings have bodies which are vulnerable to attack and easily injured. It is for this reason that all moralities have rules restricting the use of physical violence in social life. A concept like 'assault' logically could not exist unless the human body were liable to physical damage. And in more general terms principles such as 'One ought not to harm' or 'One ought to help people in distress' clearly reflect the facts that people are liable to injury and are vulnerable physically and psychologically to deliberate attacks or accidental mishaps.

Second, human needs and wants can more adequately be satisfied co-operatively, by division of labour, than by each fending for himself. These facts are reflected not only in the complexities of economic organization but also in concepts such as 'neighbourliness'.

Third, human beings are approximately equal in most respects. Some people are stronger or cleverer or more attractive than others, but on the whole these natural gifts tend to balance out, giving us all an interest in accepting principles which work for the benefit of all.

Fourth, human rationality is limited, and rules are therefore helpful to guide us on the likely consequence of action. J. S. Mill said that rules are like signposts which guide us when we are not sure where to go, or they distil the wisdom of mankind on the consequences of action.

Fifth, human sympathy exists − by nature we have the germs of benevolence or compassion within us − but our benevolence is limited and easily swamped by the stronger natural endowment of self-assertion in all its forms. We recognize this in each other and therefore have an interest in belonging to a system of morality the principles of which correct our bias towards self-interest.

Finally, the resources of the environment are scarce and require work for their production and distribution through service industries. Scarcity gives us an interest in property and the many rules for the legitimate ownership and fair transfer of property and other goods.

6. CONCLUSION

These six facts put together explain why we have an *interest* in accepting a system of morality and why morality is *desirable*. For it seems to follow from these obvious natural facts that, on the whole, we shall all do better for ourselves by belonging to a system of organization such as is provided by morality, especially when the more basic of the moral principles are enshrined in the additional system of law and safeguarded by legal sanctions.

The most basic of these principles of what we have called 'consensus morality' are the following:

1. One ought not to harm other people physically or psychologically (non-maleficence).

2. One ought to give positive help to people wherever necessary (benevolence or beneficence, and compassion).

3. One ought to treat people fairly or equally before the law, in the ownership and transfer of goods, and in rewarding labour (justice).

4. One ought to produce the best possible consequences (or the greatest happiness) for the majority (utility).

These principles can all be seen to be acceptable to human beings granted the six limitations already mentioned of their nature and situation. And, of course, these four broad principles will give rise to many detailed rules of helping others, property rules, rules of fair dealing, and many more.

Chapter 4
AUTONOMY AND RESPECT

1. FROM CONSENSUS TO MORALITY

So far we have tried to explain why we all have an *interest* in belonging to a system of morality, and why, granted our human make-up, certain consensus principles will tend to emerge. We have not so far mentioned the crucial feature of morality − that it is *authoritative*, and not just appealing or persuasive. Our question therefore is: How does a distinctively moral 'ought' emerge from the principles of consensus morality?

The answer to this question is that persuasive consensus principles become authoritative moral principles to the extent that they presuppose the supreme value of the individual human being. We shall add this to the list as:

5. One ought to respect (value) a human being above all (the principle of the autonomous person).

The principle of the autonomous person is not like the others, in that the moral authority of the others derives from it, or it is presupposed by them. If we judge the other principles to impose an 'ought' of morality as distinct from self-interest on us, then we are presupposing the authority of the principle of respect for the autonomous person.

Various questions now arise. What does it mean to be an autonomous person and what is it to 'respect' an autonomous person? How is the principle of respect for autonomy presupposed by the other principles? Are there any other basic principles in this moral system? What is the source of the moral validity of the principle of respect for autonomy itself?

To be an autonomous person is to have the ability to be able to choose for oneself or more extensively to be able to formulate and carry out one's own plans or policies. The moral importance we attach to these abilities is reflected in our approval of traits of character such as 'being able to stand on own's own two feet', 'knowing what one wants', 'having aims in own's life', or 'being able to make up own's own mind'. The connection between developing such traits of character and being a person is reflected in theories of education which stress the importance of cultivating such dispositions in children. Conversely, to impair a person's abilities to formulate and carry out aims and policies of his own devising is to that extent to injure him as a person. For example, if a person has been injured physically or mentally there is often a tendency for friends to help this person too much, for it is often easier to do something for people than to wait patiently while they try to do it for themselves; and this ease and convenience can assume the guise of kindness. But it may be a subtle way of eroding someone's nature as a person. The development of personality can also be blocked in grander ways by political arrangements which restrict the images people can form of themselves, or by consumer societies which impose certain images on people. We can call this feature of the autonomous person the ability to be self-determining.

A second feature of the autonomous person is the ability to govern one's conduct by rules or values. Kant attaches such importance to this feature that he identifies autonomy with it. For Kant, the 'autonomy of the will' is the distinctive mark of a person or a 'rational being' because he holds that it is through acts of rational choice that the highest side of human nature is expressed, but we are taking the less extreme position that autonomy is also expressed through the pursuit of desires and purposes in self-determination. Nevertheless, Kant is correct in stressing that the ability to be detached, to stand back from one's desires and mould one's conduct in terms of rules valid for others as well as oneself, is a mark of the mature person. That is why we say that the two abilities − to be self-determining and to be self-governing in terms of rules valid for all — make up the important moral concept of the autonomous person.

It should be stressed that our account of the autonomous person is not excluding as unimportant human emotions and desires. Kant's account of human nature involves a division of the person into a rational and a sentient or desiring aspect with a value judgement on the importance of the rational element. We, on the other hand, see human nature as a unity. Reason and desire are both clearly involved in the exercise of self-determination, since our desires, needs, and wants suggest our aims, and reason suggests the means to attain them.

Even in self-governing, reason and emotion are both involved. Kant thinks of desires and emotions as wayward and arbitrary causal forces determining action, and he therefore understands the self-governing processes entirely in terms of reason, and uses a legal analogy of 'self-legislation'. Hume, on the other hand, holds that reason on its own is dead and inert and cannot lead to action, so he sees the process of self-governing in terms of the exercise of a 'calm passion'. Now certainly Hume is correct in stressing that there is an emotional side to the calmness and detachment of some aspects of morality, but on the other hand Kant is correct in thinking of a moral situation as one which involves the use of practical reason. One cannot be calm and open to relevant scientific or other facts without the appropriate stabilizing emotions, but equally emotions require to be informed and decisions generalized by reason. In both self-determination and self-government, then, there is a unity of reason and emotion.

Indeed, even in the experience of emotion itself reason is involved. For emotions in their characteristic human form are not just physiologically-based sensations but have an essential rational core. For example, to experience anger or resentment or love is to *see* a situation *as* having certain features, and to have inappropriate emotions is to stress the wrong features of a situation or to deny the existence of the relevant ones. In the process of dying, for instance, the problem can sometimes be that of persuading or enabling the patient to see certain features of his condition which he is denying. For example, he may believe that his increasing weakness is to be blamed on the ment he is receiving and that a change of drugs or consultant reverse this trend. Relatives may encourage this false belief. in, relatives may believe that there is hope for someone who is still breathing with the help of a ventilator even although he is brain-dead or in a permanent vegetative state. Only by having an objective or rational awareness of his situation can the patient or relatives be brought to acceptance and the experience of appropriate emotion.

The autonomous person in his/her self-determination, self-governing and emotional reactions is a unity and, as we shall now go on to argue, the morally appropriate treatment of an autonomous person ought to be determined by awareness of this unified human nature.

2. RESPECT AND OTHER PRINCIPLES

To *respect* a person as an autonomous being, or, in Kant's phrase, to respect a person as an end, is to take into account in one's conduct that he/she has an autonomous nature, that he/she is self-determining and self-governing, or that he/she has desires, feelings and reason. To 'take this into account' is to employ the four moral principles already mentioned. These were the principles of non-maleficence, benevolence, or compassion, justice or fairness, and utility. It should begin to emerge now why these are morally appropriate ways of treating autonomous persons. In so far as people are self-determining the most appropriate way of treating them will most often be leaving them alone − not harming them but respecting their liberty. But sometimes plans and projects go wrong and then benevolence might become appropriate − the offering of positive help and assistance. This can range from the trivial directing of a lost stranger to his destination or the holding open of a shop door for an overburdened shopper, to the gift of millions of pounds by a philanthropist to a charity. Obviously all the caring professions are frequently governed by this moral principle, but perhaps in its application to the caring professions the moral principle in question is better described by the term 'compassion'. What exactly is involved in compassion, or benevolence, in a health care context?

First of all the natural ingredients, as it were, of compassion are part of the make-up of a normal human being. We all have the capacity to feel with others, to enter to some extent into their predicament and share their emotions. This capacity is displayed even in an extreme situation, for it is the basis of the strategy for dealing with terrorists who have taken hostages, namely to delay doing anything as long as possible on the grounds that it is emotionally difficult to kill hostages if you have shared experiences with them. This capacity to identify with the feelings of others is the natural basis of compassion.

Compassion, however, is not just a matter of feeling with others — it is not just passive. To have compassion is to be moved to act on the basis of the promptings of natural emotion. We prefer the old-fashioned term 'compassion' to the semi-technical term 'empathy' on the grounds that the latter suggests something passive. All caring workers must attempt to develop in themselves the capacity for feeling with others, but compassion, like benevolence, requires an active response. In a similar way, the term 'sympathy' is ambiguous as between passive and active modes of expression. If someone is described as 'very sympathetic' this might mean simply that he shared one's feelings, or that he went on to do something about one's predicament. To be compassionate, however, requires both responses.

There is also a cognitive side to compassion which we have already described in our account of understanding in Chapter 2. In that account we spoke of 'vertical' understanding, of imaginative insight into a particular person's situation, which differs from a social science understanding of *types* of case, such as 'the elderly patient'. To be an 'understanding person' is to have a biographer's or historian's flair for seeing just how this patient is where he is, *coupled with* compassion. Indeed, in health care the imaginative insight cannot exist without the compassion.

A different and most important point about compassion emerges if we compare it with pity. Pity is like the passive mode of sympathy, but pity can involve a certain condescension to its objects. But it is vital to remember that the objects of compassion in health care are typically autonomous persons. (We shall deal later with comatose or incompetent patients.) Pity therefore is inappropriate to the dignity of the autonomous person, especially with its overtones of paternalism. Compassion then is the term we have chosen to characterize the mode of dealing with autonomous persons who have experienced ill-health or other misfortune: it involves emotion, positive help, and imaginative understanding, but is tempered by the awareness of its objects.

The third principle involved in respect is that of justice or fairness. This is a wide principle applying to the legal and political as well as the moral sphere. As far as its moral side is concerned the principle applies first to our dealings with one person or group as compared with others. This is sometimes called 'distributive justice', and can be expressed in the form 'You ought to treat like cases alike'. The point here is not that it is necessarily wrong to discriminate in favour of or against other people or groups, but rather that any such discrimination must be justified; the presumption is for equality of treatment in like cases and the onus of justification is on the discriminator to justify his bias. For example, if two people require renal dialysis then the presumption is that they should be treated alike, but perhaps one has more utility to the community as a whole, or has been promised treatment, and can therefore justifiably be preferred to the other, if the resource is scarce.

Justice has another side to it, concerned with treating individuals rightly in the light of their own wants, needs and merits. For example, if a doctor is withholding the truth about a patient's condition, a colleague or a relative might say, 'I don't think you are being *fair* to him, he asked to be told the truth.' Justice or fairness in this sense is sometimes expressed by the concept of 'deserts'. For example, we might say 'He deserves better care than he got.'

But whether in the form of just distribution of goods or just deserts, the concept of justice is clearly connected with the autonomous person and with a proper respect for him. We are all equal as autonomous persons and the respect due to autonomy is due to or deserved by each individual autonomous person alike.

We have spoken of respect as a supreme *principle* and of subordinate *principles* such as non-maleficence, benevolence, and justice through which it is expressed. But compassion fits uneasily into the category of the principle since it necessarily refers, as we have seen, both to a standard of acting and also to a mode of *feeling*. This raises the question of the concept of respect itself. Is it basically a principle − we even described it as a supreme principle − or what? The answer is that basically it is an *attitude*, although an attitude which gives rise to principles. Having the attitude of respect towards autonomous persons, a moral agent can adopt the principles of non-maleficence, benevolence, or compassion, as is appropriate. The appropriate principle will, as it were, crystallize out of the attitude of respect and form round the situations in which people may find themselves.

It is arguable that an attitude so constituted may best be described as one of love. Many different kinds of attitude may be called 'love' but the relevant kind seems to be what in the language of the Gospels is called *agape*. The term *agape* is not without its own obscurities but it seems the most suitable for characterizing an attitude which combines a regard for others as self-governing with a compassion for them in their pursuit of ends. It is an attitude illustrated in the story of the Good Samaritan, and again in the well-known passage from St John's Gospel: 'Greater love hath no man than this, that a man lay down his life for his friends.' To lay down own's life for one's friends may be a supreme example of making the ends of others one's own, but it should also be noted that to *accept* such sacrifice may also be to show respect or *agape* because such acceptance may be an expression of the recognition that others too are moral agents who can follow moral rules and display the attitude of *agape* in their lives.

How does the principle of utility fit into this? Not so neatly, it must be admitted. The principle of utility tells us that we ought to seek the best possible consequences, or the greatest happiness, for the greater number of people. In other words, utility is not concerned with individuals but with majorities, with aggregates. It is what might be regarded as a principle for administrators or legislators. Indeed, it was developed in the nineteenth century as a theory highlighting the need for the reform of the criminal code. In the version of the theory which has become accepted — rule-utilitarianism as opposed to act-utilitarianism — it is the utility of policies, classes of action, rules of behaviour rather than of individual actions which is stressed. It is therefore a principle of particular relevance to health care managers. Nevertheless, there can be no sense in promoting the interests or happiness of aggregates of people unless one is already presupposing the supreme value of the persons who make up these aggregates. The principle of utility can therefore be seen as an administrative expression of respect. It would be wrong however to conceal the conflict which can break out between justice, treating like cases alike, and utility, treating some groups or even individuals better than others for the believed good of the majority. We shall illustrate this in later chapters.

3. SELF-DEVELOPMENT AND THE VIRTUES

We have so far been discussing the other-regarding principles and attitudes of morality. Let us now turn to the question of the self-regarding aspects. Some philosophers deny that there can be a self-regarding side to morality, for they see morality as having an essentially social function, concerned only with regulating one's conduct *vis-à-vis* other members of society. Such a view has developed out of one strand in J. S. Mill's thinking. Mill in his essay *On Liberty* seemed to be arguing that moral issues arise only to the extent that one's conduct harms other people; in so far as one's conduct affects only oneself it does not raise a moral issue. Yet in the same work, Mill has a chapter on 'self-development' and does not seem to regard it as a matter of moral indifference what kind of person one is. As he puts it, 'It really is of importance not only what men do, but also what manner of men they are that do it.'* And this view, that there are moral duties to cultivate in oneself certain characteristic human excellences, goes back to Plato and Aristotle and is taken up in a slightly different form by the Judaeo-Christian traditions. According to these traditions we have our nature in trust from our Creator and have therefore a duty to cultivate the talents we have in trust. For Kant the principle (or attitude) which we state in the form 'One ought to respect autonomous persons' takes the form 'Respect human nature, whether in your own person or in that of another.' In other words, Kant makes ample room for the idea of a self-regarding area of morality.

This is an important area of morality for those in the caring professions, and it is the more important in that its neglect can seem a virtue. It is quite common for professional carers to live a life of devotion to their patients as a result of which their own lives become empty and impoverished. They have cultivated only their medical knowledge and skills and have nothing to say on anything else.

The duty of self-development can also be justified in terms of its benefit to other people. Since so much of the success of a doctor, nurse, dentist, or other health worker depends on the relationship each has with a patient, and since the nature of that relationship depends partly on the patient's perceptions of his helper, it is vital that the professional should be seen as an authentic human being who happens to be a doctor, nurse, or other carer. If a doctor is to give himself to others he must have something to give! We have argued in Chapter 2 that there is a moral element in the most technical-seeming medical or nursing judgements. If that is so, then it is important that these judgements should be the products not just of a technical, scientific mind, but of a humane and compassionate one. That is why it is important for the health care professional to be *more* than just that; to be a morally developed person who happens to follow a given professional path. Self-development, then, is good both for its own sake and for what it gives to patients, friends and families.

*Mill, J. S. *On Liberty*, Chapter 3.

4. JUSTIFYING ULTIMATE PRINCIPLES

We have asserted that the ultimate principle (or attitude) of morality can be expressed in the form 'One ought to respect human nature (or autonomy) whether in one's own person or in that of another person.' Can this be justified?

The question is ambiguous. First of all, it might mean: How can we justify the claim that all moral principles are ultimately reducible to or analysable in terms of the principle of respect for persons? This question is answerable, but not briefly. We have already tried to show how principles such as non-maleficence, benevolence, compassion, justice and utility are expressions of respect, and in Part 2 we shall try to show how more specific rules, such as 'One ought to tell the truth' are also expressions of respect. We shall also consider and answer objections to this claim in our next chapter. For example, there are the problems which arise when the patient is not a person in the sense so far outlined − where there is mental handicap or senility, where young children are involved, where patients are kept alive by ventilators, and where the status of embryos is questioned. We shall take these problems as they come, but maintain in advance that our ultimate principle is still the operative one, although the attitude of respect must always be moulded by the nature of what is respected.

There is a second level to the question of justification. How do we know that our principle is *true?* It is just a matter of taste or opinion or Western prejudice? This is a fundamental question of moral philosophy, but let us briefly review some answers. One answer is that of the reductionist, who aims to explain moral principles in terms of something else, for example, pleasure, or God's commands. This answer still leaves us with questions such as: Why ought we to obey God's commands? or: Is all pleasure really morally good? In other words, morality has slipped out of the new formula and remains unjustified. A second answer is a conventionalist one. Granted that we can explain subsidiary moral principles in terms of respect for persons, it is just a convention or axiom that it is itself taken to be ultimate. Just as there can be various logically coherent systems of geometry, each turning on its own axioms and postulates, so in morality we have been exploring one possible system in which respect for persons is axiomatic. The trouble with this approach is that morality may require one's life and one's all, and it seems odd to make such sacrifices for a convention or axiom; it would be rational simply to adopt another convention. By contrast, an ultimate principle, one wants to say, is *true*.

A third answer given by some philosophers, often called intuitionists, is that one can just 'see' or intuit that the principle is ultimately valid. The trouble here is in analysing the sense of intuition involved and in showing why someone's intuition can validate an ultimate principle.

Perhaps the way ahead is to turn to a fourth and more modest sense of justification. We do all make moral judgements like 'It is unfair to keep the truth from him' or 'That was unkind'. Such moral judgements are common, and if we analyse them they can be shown (as we have tried to show) to have implicit in them the ultimate principle of respect; they would not be authoritative without this principle. To 'justify' a system of morality, then, is first to articulate in detail the systematic connections which obtain among its concepts and the function it has in a total way of life, and then, secondly, to identify the principle which makes it authoritative for those sharing that way of life.

But why is it authoritative for those sharing the way of life? The most plausible answer to this question takes us to the third stage in justification. It is authoritative because it is just the case that we are so made, or our human natures have so developed, that we accept this principle as authoritative; we cannot help presupposing it in our dealing with other people. Whether this feature of our human nature is best explained in terms of socio-biology, deep-rooted cultural conditioning, or divine creation can be left open. It may seem that this three-tier kind of justification is a poor substitute for some grander metaphysical sort, but if the latter is not possible we must make do with what is.

5. DEONTOLOGY AND RIGHTS

By way of a postscript we note that many books on professional ethics include discussions of 'deontology' and 'rights'. For the sake of completeness, we shall indicate how these terms fit into our argument. The theory of deontology is most accurately placed as a theory critical of utilitarianism. Whereas the utilitarian holds that all duties are justifiable in terms of their consequences, the deontologist is said to hold that none or only some are justifiable in that way. For certain other duties, such as truth-telling, promise-keeping, and justice, no utilitarian justification is possible; they are just ultimate duties. We are thus left by the deontologist with a *number* of ultimate principles, stating that certain sorts of action are *just right* in themselves, or are just duties.

Our view is that the deontologist is correct in the negative part of his theory, that is, his criticism of utilitarianism, but likewise the utilitarian is correct in pointing out that the deontologist leaves us with a heap of duties unrelated to each other and to good states of affairs in the world. We hope we have shown that what is presupposed in our judgements about the moral importance of, say, truth-telling or acting fairly is the autonomous person. Moreover, utilitarianism, while it is a neater theory than deontology, does not explain why the happiness of the majority is desirable. We hope therefore to have the edge on both.

Many philosophers express their theories in terms of rights. We shall also occasionally use this expression. But the vocabulary of rights is simply an alternative way of expressing what we have put in terms of principles. Rights are created by rules or principles, and therefore moral rights are one way of expressing moral principles.

6. CONCLUSION

This chapter has been concerned with the way in which the consensus principles which help social life to proceed in a more harmonious and co-operative way become authoritative moral principles when they are seen to be presupposing the supreme value of the individual and therefore the attitude of respect for the autonomous person. Morality can be seen as having three dimensions:

	Principles	
3rd person social morality of majorities and aggregates	Utility Justice	
2nd person face-to-face morality of personal encounters	Non-maleficence Compassion (benevolence) Justice	Respect for the autonomous individual
1st person self-referring morality of authenticity, integrity	Self-development	

Chapter 5

EMBRYOS, PERSONS, AND OTHER HUMAN BEINGS

In our account of the autonomous person and the attitude which is morally appropriate to autonomous persons we have been assuming that we are dealing with mature and rational adults. But this is often not the case in health care, where the patient or client may be a baby, perhaps even an embryo, a dementing elderly person, a mentally handicapped adult, or someone in a coma. How do these categories fit into the analysis of the previous chapter?

There is no one type of answer to that question. These various cases differ from the standard case of the rational adult in different ways, and there are no sharp lines between the deviant and the standard cases. Nevertheless, at the risk of question-begging, we shall group these situations in certain ways. In one group we shall place the embryo and also the patient with irreversible brain damage being kept breathing on a ventilator. The discussion of these situations raises questions such as: When does human life begin, and when does it cease? Is it ever right to carry out experiments on an embryo and, if so, until what stage in its development? We shall here make some philosophical points about these questions, and discuss some practical implications in Part 2.

A second group of questions arises about people suffering from mental handicap, mental disturbance, senility, and also about young children. Do they differ in morally significant ways from the rational adult and, if so, does that mean they are not due the respect accorded to autonomous persons? Can they be meaningfully said to give informed consent to their treatment and, if not, what safeguards can they have? How do we understand their behaviour?

We shall discuss these two groups of problems separately, although they raise overlapping issues, and we shall return to them again in Part 2.

1. LIFE AS A MORAL PHENOMENON

We have made the central moral principle of health care that of respect for the autonomous individual. But for many people the central moral question is: When does life begin? For them the answer to that question determines when respect ought to be shown. Those who ask that question are often prepared to answer it by saying that life begins at conception, and draw from that view the implications that abortion is always or often morally wrong, and that experiments on embryos, no matter how early in their development, are always wrong because they are experiments on what is at least potentially a human being.

The assessment of their argument is a complex matter. If we take it in a biological sense it is simply not true that life begins at conception. In the biological sense life is a constantly evolving process and conception is only one stage in such a process. It is a stronger claim to say that life begins to matter from the moral point of view at conception. But note that this is not a scientific claim − there are no scientific facts, present or future, which determine 'when life begins' if that means 'when life begins to have moral significance'; for scientific facts cannot logically determine moral judgements. Assuming that it is a moral and not a scientific judgement that life matters morally at conception we can now ask whether it is a well-founded moral judgement.

Our argument in favour of the view that life matters morally at conception is that the fertilized egg has the complete genetic material of the adult and therefore can be considered a potential adult, even a potential specific adult. Consequently, it can be vested with at least some of the rights of the adult human being, and certainly the right to be allowed to develop that potentiality.

There are two weaknesses in potentiality arguments of this sort.* The first is that it does not follow from the fact that something is potentially an X that it should be allowed, encouraged, or assisted to become an X. An acorn is potentially an oak, but it does not follow that it should be allowed, encouraged, or assisted to become an oak. The strength of this point in the human case is dramatically brought out if we consider that in the very weak sense in which a fertilized egg is potentially a mature person, an unfertilized egg is potentially a fertilized one − in each case the potentiality will be fulfilled if, but only if, a large number of events which might or might not take place do actually take place. For example, if we are dealing with the unfertilized egg, then its potentiality as a fertilized egg is realized if a male fertilizes it. But we do not regard it as a duty on males to fertilize all the eggs they can! In a similar way there is no duty to enable or assist the fertilized egg to realize its potentiality as a mature person.

The second weakness is that it does not follow from the fact that something is potentially an X that we should treat it as if it were now an X. We are all potentially 20 years older than we presently are − indeed we are potentially dead − but we ought not now to be treated as if we were. Thus the fact (if it is one) that a fertilized egg is potentially an adult human being does not give grounds for investing the egg with any of the rights of the adult. This is not to say that as human genetic material it has no moral significance at all.

The way forward may be to change the question. We have been asking: Does the fertilized egg have moral significance or not? Perhaps a better question might be: *How much* moral significance does it have? In answering the latter question we can assume that there is a continuance of development from conception, and that our moral attitudes to the embryo should be moulded by its stage of development. The moral significance of the fertilized egg will not be a large one, but in recognition that it does have some moral significance, the Warnock Committee

*These weaknesses are well discussed in Harris, J. (1985). *The Value of Life*. Routledge & Kegan Paul, London, especially Chapter 1.

suggested that experiments should be carried out only by properly licensed bodies and only during the first 14 days.

Moral attitudes to the embryo become much more important with the development of the brain and the central nervous system (CNS), which create the possibility of the experiences of pain and perhaps some elementary sensory cognition. Killing an embryo at this stage is clearly a much more serious matter than killing it at a few days. We shall raise some questions about abortion in Part 2. The possibility of independent existence (viability) is another important stage in the acquisition of moral rights. Birth is yet another stage and later still, in early childhood, come possibilities for acquiring independent plans and purposes, then self-consciousness and finally the autonomy which we have noted in our previous chapter as the distinctive feature of the adult human being.

It is important to note here that an important stage, according to this analysis, is the development of the brain and CNS. This criterion is derived from another area of morally controversial medicine − resuscitation and keeping alive on ventilators. In this area of medicine it is often asked: When is a person really dead? A widely accepted answer seems to be that the death of a person is to be equated with brain death or brainstem death, and that what is kept alive by a ventilator is not a person but a body. We have extracted this criterion and applied it to the beginning of life; when there is a functioning brain and CNS there is a beginning to distinctively human life, and life at this stage begins to matter morally in a strong sense.

To summarize, then, the view we are rejecting is that at conception there is a person or even, in any significant sense, a potential person. Hence, we do not hold that the development of the embryo is the development *of* a person. We find it more plausible to hold that the embryo develops gradually *into* a person. It does not follow from this that there are no duties to non-persons. What does follow is that a being should be respected for the sort of being it is: living human tissue, an embryo with a brain and CNS, an embryo capable of independent existence, a child with plans of its own and self-consciousness, and finally a fully autonomous adult.

2. ARGUMENTS FOR RESUSCITATION

It might be said that whereas a brain-dead patient on a ventilator is dead, there are cases of patients in a coma whose brains are not dead. These patients, it is often argued, should be maintained on life-support systems unless or until 'brain death' can be established. Equally, this argument refers to the absolute requirement to resuscitate any person whose respiration suddenly ceases, as again, brain death cannot be assumed at that particular moment.

Arguments to support this position are essentially based on three different moral assumptions. The first of these holds that the *basis* of a decision to resuscitate or not to do so will always be *uncertain*, or *subjective*, or *irrelevant*. It will be *uncertain* if the basis for the decision is sought in scientific or medical 'facts' such as a poor prognosis, for how certain can one be of these 'facts'? An extreme version of this position is that even if the patient appears to be dead, criteria for death are too controversial to be given credence in these circumstances. It is likely that doctors can make mistakes and an unforeseen turn of events may occur, including what religious minded people might call a miracle.

The basis will be *subjective* if it is an assessment of the potential quality of life for the person who is or is not to be resuscitated, for any assessment of quality of life will always be a subjective assessment on the part of the health care team. If the basis for the decision not to resuscitate is that the provisions for resuscitation and the continued care of the comatose patient are too expensive, then this is held to be *irrelevant* by those arguing for resuscitation in all instances.

The force of all three points concerning the *basis* of a decision not to resuscitate can be exaggerated. We have ourselves in Chapter 2 discussed the uncertainties of applying medical science to particular cases, but very often the scientific facts can be established beyond reasonable doubt. We shall deal with quality of life and with the economics of health care in Part 2, but can say here that assessment of quality of life is not entirely subjective. There are some human qualities, like having a functioning brain, or being more than a vegetable, that must be assumed in any account of quality of life, and when they are absent the case for not resuscitating is overwhelming. Again, we discuss the economics for health care in Part 2, but it is one of our assumptions that economics is not irrelevant to the morality of health care; resources diverted to X are at the expense of resources for Y. The case for diverting resources to X must therefore be made if the decision to do so is to be morally sound, and it is difficult to make out a case for the continued care of comatose patients.

The second assumption holds that although the scientific or economic basis for rejecting resuscitation may be sound, the *decision* not to resuscitate is always from various points of view wrong in itself. One point of view is that of those who hold a fundamentalist religious position about the sanctity of all forms of human life. This line occasionally merges into that of the doctor's inherent or sacred duty to maintain life at all costs. Failing to maintain life at all costs, it might be said, would be negating the very essence of being a doctor.

Complementary to this argument we can appeal to the rights of the patient. If the doctor *qua* doctor has a duty to maintain life so also we can say that the patient *qua* patient has a right to treatment, in this case resuscitation.

In assessing such arguments we encounter the impossibility of convincing those who are deeply committed to religious positions. However, it should be pointed out that whatever may be true of Buddhism, the Judaeo-Christian tradition is not one stressing the sanctity of *life*, but one stressing the creation of man in the image of God. It is the person who is sacred, not the corrupt body. There is no mandate in the Scriptures for maintaining the body on a ventilator.

The associated arguments, that the doctor *qua* doctor has a duty to maintain life at all costs, and that the patient *qua* patient has a right to receive treatment at all costs, are seriously confused. In the first place, the definition offered of the role of doctor − to maintain life − is one-sided, and there is no reason to accept it any more than other definitions often mentioned, such as that the doctor by definition relieves suffering. In the second place, nothing of any moral substance follows from a definition, whether of doctor or patient (see pp. 122–3).

The third type of argument for the view that we ought always to resuscitate comes from those who concede that, while the basis for the decision not to resuscitate may be sound, and that the decision itself may not be intrinsically wrong, the *consequences* of such decisions are always bad. There are various ways in which consequences may be invoked. First, it might be said that public awareness that doctors do not always resuscitate may undermine confidence in the profession. Second, the 'slippery slope' argument may be used in this context. If particular kinds of patient are 'allowed' to die today who will it be tomorrow? A third extension of this fear of generalizing consequences is expressed in the suggestion that patients who are identified as not to be resuscitated may generally receive less attention and care than if they were not so labelled. A fourth consequentialist argument refers to the role of the family. If a doctor tries to share responsibility for the decision not to resuscitate with the patient's family, they may be likely to decide so for the wrong reasons, for their own rather than the patient's interest. If, on the other hand, the family agree to non-intervention for what appear to be good reasons, they may still be left with lifelong guilt or doubt about whether they have acted in the right way.

None of these arguments for resuscitation is wholly convincing. The public confidence argument cuts both ways. Even if it were true that some members of the public become anxious if they believe that comatose patients are not always resuscitated other members of the public are relieved to hear that this is so, for there is sometimes a fear that comatose patients are officiously resuscitated when they and their relatives might wish that they should be allowed to die with dignity. Again, the 'slippery slope' argument, like all uses of it (see pp. 129–30) is effective only if we have good reason for believing that there is a slope and that it is slippery.

The third and fourth arguments are stronger. There is clearly a psychological danger that nursing staff, knowing that a patient is not to be resuscitated, will not give attentive nursing care. This is a danger, but one which nursing staff can guard against. Families should clearly be consulted and counselled, but there is no need to suppose that for any sinister reason the medical staff will concur in a family wish for no resuscitation unless this is medically indicated.

In addition to the three types of argument we have considered for always resuscitating the comatose patient there is another which is sometimes invoked here and more generally − the argument that there is a morally significant difference between acts and omissions. If someone is on a respirator it might be said to be morally worse to switch it off − thus doing something to kill him − than it would be to omit to put him on it in the first place.

Acts and omissions arguments − like slippery slope arguments − have different strengths in different contexts. In this context the argument is weak because it depends for its force on the probability of death. But the probability of death is just as great when we omit to switch on the ventilator as it is when we switch it off. From this moral perspective it seems to make no difference.

The moral dilemmas of the health care team can be greatly eased by the existence of a 'living will'. Sometimes people record their wishes on the matter of resuscitation. Such expressions of preference may have no legal force but they obviously assist in the solution of moral problems on this matter. The use of such documents should be encouraged as medicine advances in its technical possibilities.

In discussing the development of the embryo we mentioned that it was not the development *of* a person but development *into* a person by living human tissue. The conclusion of this section is that as the brain decays we have a degeneration *out of* a person back into living human tissue, and then back into the dust and ashes from which we came. A human being should be respected during this process, but at a certain point in it the appropriate sort of respect is not the same as that for an autonomous person but the sort we might have for human tissue. It is a separate question, although of the first importance in morality, that the feelings of friends and relatives are also involved, and that they must be consulted about any policy of removing organs. A 'living will' − kidney card or the like − would again give guidance.

In summary, we have been considering the objection that the basic moral principle of health care is not 'respect for the autonomous person' but 'respect for the sanctity of life'. This kind of objection can be pressed acutely in the context of the debate as to when the comatose patient should or should not be resuscitated. We are not persuaded by any arguments for resuscitation unless it can be shown that there is a reasonable chance that the patient will, when resuscitated, have the prospect of a life with a certain quality − a quality which is at least on the margins of autonomy. Otherwise death with dignity seems morally indicated.

3. LESS THAN A PERSON?

In analysing the nature of the mature and rational adult we said that he was self-determining and self-governing, and we described the attitude of respect and stated the principles to which it gives rise. If we try to apply this analysis to a mentally handicapped person we run into difficulties. For example, we do not feel that we should necessarily accede to his wishes, far less assist him to attain his objectives, if we believe that what the person intends is likely to harm him. It might be said that the same is true of the mentally competent person. But the all-important difference is that in the case of a rational adult we can consult him and draw attention to the risks or drawbacks of a given project, whereas in the case of the more severely mentally handicapped person, a senile patient or a young child, we cannot always be sure that he understands his situation, and therefore we ought not to allow him an entirely free hand in deciding his actions. The possible inability to understand is of course a matter of degree, but it may be reasonable to say that in extreme cases those without full measure of the 'distinctive endowment' of a human being *ought* not to be given the same sort of treatment accorded to a rational adult.

There is another side to this. We have claimed that benevolence and compassion are essential components of the attitude of respect accorded to the autonomous person, but we have also pointed out that sometimes we should stand aside and *allow* such a person to pursue his aims in his own way; it can be officious, patronizing, interfering, or possessive to be 'helpful' in every instance. But in the case of a mentally handicapped person, the temptation to 'help' can be overpowering. This is particularly the case in families, where there can be a strong identification with the mentally handicapped person and where 'pity' can become a morally inferior substitute for compassion. Indeed, the desire to 'help' can overpower the legitimate claims of other members of the family and work to their detriment as well as to that of the mentally handicapped person. Again, we are dealing with matters of degree, and there is no way of drawing a clear theoretical line between the 'benevolence' which is a proper component in the attitude of respect, and the 'pity' which may become its pathological substitute and destroy it.

This ambivalence in the attitude of respect is a logical reflection of the ambivalence in the status of its object. Sometimes the word 'person' is used − in ordinary speech as much as in philosophical literature − to mark off those human beings who have the full complement of mental capabilities. It is consequently less appropriate for those who lack some or all of these capacities. The word 'person' is used in this evaluative way when we say of a senile old man that he is no longer a person: 'There isn't a person there any more', or we say of someone severely mentally ill, 'You can't at present regard him as a person at all', or we say of an infant, 'He's not really a person yet'.

On the other hand, we sometimes object to this and feel intuitively that the old or the mentally handicapped are being denigrated by this terminology, that they are being regarded as lacking something of *moral* value because they lack some *natural* capacities. This reaction is often based on a misunderstanding. The claim that a human being is not a 'person' in the semi-technical sense and is therefore not entitled to full 'respect' in the correlative technical sense, does not entail that he should be treated badly, or disregarded, or in any avoidable way made to suffer. Yet, there may be something more than an emotional reaction behind the resistance that some people experience – perhaps those especially who are involved in caring for the mentally handicapped – when they are told that their patients or clients, and particularly their children, are not fully 'persons' and are therefore not entitled to 'respect' in the full sense.

One way of identifying the legitimate source of this resistance is to compare it to our moral attitudes to animals, which is largely expressed in the principle that it is wrong to cause needless suffering. But this principle cannot wholly be accounted for by referring to animal sentience; there is another important factor. Consider, for example, the repugnance that some people feel at the spectacle of the caged lion, or the over-fed poodle trimmed into a fashionable shape, and contrast such repugnance with the approval some people feel at the well-trained sheep-dog. The point is not that the caged or pampered animal is necessarily suffering – in many cases it may well be much better off than in the wild state and show no tendency to return to it. It is rather that its animal nature is not being respected in that it is being subjected to purposes foreign to it. In a similar way, a slave may well prefer to remain in a condition of slavery, but we still feel that there is something morally wrong with the state of affairs which leads him to concur in his slavery. And so, too, many people's moral attitude to the higher animals is moulded by their awareness that animals are used as means to further human ends. This factor, along with their sentience, seems to constitute our moral attitude to animals. It is therefore possible to maintain that we have moral duties to animals (duties which, as in the case of children, for example, are made easier to perform by the existence of non-moral attitudes such as affection and pity) and that these are to be explained by the idea of respect for the type of personality in question.

Applying the same idea to mentally handicapped people we can say that they retain a certain *dignity*, and the morally appropriate attitude to them must be one of respect and cannot therefore on all occasions be simply a regard for their sentience alone. But sometimes it is the latter, and there is therefore an ambivalence in our moral attitude.

4. UNDERSTANDING MENTALLY HANDICAPPED PEOPLE

Some of the points we have made about our ambivalence of attitude to mentally handicapped or senile people can be developed, if we look at the ways in which we can explain and understand the actions of those in these categories. In the case of our understanding of fully rational persons we are assisted (as we argued in Chapter 2) both by the explanatory patterns of the social sciences and by our own intuitive and sympathetic insights. If we apply this analysis of explanation and understanding to the case of the mentally handicapped person, we find uncertainties and ambiguities. First of all, the behaviour patterns are not of the same kinds as those of a fully rational person. Second, it is harder in relation to mentally handicapped people for the fully competent person to have the sympathetic insight, the *verstehen*, into what it is like to be on the inside of such behaviour patterns. The problems and uncertainties which thus arise in applying this model of understanding to the behaviour of the mentally handicapped encourage the use of a totally different sort of model (and one which is incompatible with the attitude of respect as we have described it), and this is the causal model of understanding.

The causal model of understanding incorporates the assumption that what people do is not, despite appearance, freely chosen by them but is governed by forces and factors over which they have no control. Thus one may say to oneself, 'She can't help lashing out at me like that, she's experiencing the change of life', or 'He obviously would marry very young, he's from a broken home', appealing not to any rational thought on the agent's part but to underlying causal factors seen as explaining the action. Instead of reacting spontaneously with hostility or disapproval as would be appropriate towards a person who is responsible for his actions, a stance of detachment is taken up based on the idea that

'Of course, he can't help it'. We are tempted in ordinary life to do this to avoid the strain of fully 'reactive' encounters with other people.

Health care workers are particularly prone to the temptation to adopt this latter kind of 'objective' attitude. For example, some social workers are apt to construe everything done by a client as manifesting the workings of subconscious complexes of one kind or another; others, of a different persuasion, see what he does as manifestations of alienation, of the class struggle. Again, doctors or nurses tend to say 'You only want to do that because you see things in that way while you're ill. When you're well, you'll see things quite differently.' In both cases the effect is to undercut the reasons the agent himself would give for his action or thought and replace them by mechanisms on which the caring worker is an expert. The motivation for doing this may be, as in private life, the wish to avoid reactive encounters. But the caring worker may have no ulterior motive and may simply believe that he knows more about his client than he himself can do. In either case, the implication is that the client is not to be regarded as a self-determining being who acts in pursuance of his own purposes.

It might be objected that if we assume such attitudes to be wrong we are begging the question against determinism, which is after all a widely held position. But this is not the case, for many determinists also would wish to reject an analysis of human action which made no reference to the wishes and purposes of the individual agent, and depicted him, not just as determined but also as governed by forces outside his conscious control. Even those determinists who think that some forms of determinism can be reconciled with moral responsibility would have to admit that *this* form cannot be so reconciled.

It might be objected that we are talking about people who are mentally handicapped and who are therefore governed to a more than average extent by non-rational factors. In these cases at least, whatever is to be said about 'normal' cases, we are surely dealing with people for whom a detached, 'objective' attitude is correct, as it would be for the psychiatrist dealing with someone who is mentally disturbed. Now it cannot be denied that there is something in this argument, but several points must be noted in qualification of it. For example, there is always a temptation to extend this kind of attitude beyond those people, or those aspects of people, which would justify it. The temptation is there because this kind of objective attitude is often the easier option, and can indeed seem more 'professional'. But its adoption, where it is discovered by the recipient, or vaguely 'sensed', is hurtful, because the person is made to feel (what is indeed the case) that he is not being taken seriously as a person. In other words, this kind of attitude, correlated with the attempt to see behaviour in causal terms, is incompatible with the moral attitude of *respect*, although it is compatible with pity. It can also be added that the policy of treating people as rational unless proved otherwise may have the effect of fostering rationality, which is not an all-or-nothing matter.

It is indeed the phrase 'not all-or-nothing' which constitutes the whole difficulty. If the behaviour of the mentally handicapped were either fully appropriate or not appropriate for causal explanation the theoretical difficulties would disappear. But since there are degrees of mental handicap, there are problems about the appropriate moral attitude and problems about what sort of understanding is appropriate, whether the sympathetic appreciation of how behaviour fits into patterns of familiar purposes, or the causal understanding we might have when, for example, there are biochemical bases for behaviour disorders. There is therefore an ineradicable ambivalence in our attitudes to the mentally handicapped and similar categories of people.

5. CONCLUSION

In this chapter we have been examining the moral attitudes which are appropriate for human beings — and, indeed, for animals — who do not fully embody the capacities of the autonomous adult. There are cases of many different sorts involved: the embryo at conception, babies, dementing adults, comatose patients, human beings with ranging degrees of mental handicap. The conclusion which has emerged is that autonomy is not an all-or-nothing matter, and that correlatively the attitude of respect must vary depending on its object. The full respect due to the mature autonomous adult is not appropriate for the dementing elderly human being or the mentally handicapped, although elements in that attitude are appropriate. At the one extreme, that of the early days of conception, the respect is simply the minimum due to live human tissue, and at the other extreme we pay our last respects to the dignity of a former person by switching off the ventilator. Nothing in all this forces us to abandon our basic moral principle in favour of one stressing above all other considerations the sanctity of life.

Chapter 6

INDIVIDUAL AND GROUP
RESPONSIBILITY

1. THE SENSES OF 'RESPONSIBLE'

The autonomous person, we said, was self-determining and
self-governing, and in Chapter 5 we considered some difficult
and borderline cases. In this chapter we shall look at another
aspect of autonomous persons, namely that they can be held
responsible for what they do. There are various sides to this. For
example, in all health care professions we find hierarchical types
of organization. The junior doctor is responsible *to* seniors *for*
the performance of various duties, and likewise the junior nurse
is responsible to senior nurses for the performance of various
duties, and all are responsible to employers, and in another sense
to their professions, and to the general public for the exercise of
their various skills. To the extent that they are responsible they
can be praised for excellence in the discharge of their duties or
blamed as negligent or deficient in various ways. Clearly, then,
the concept of responsibility is a complex one and we shall begin
by noting in a more systematic way the basic senses of the term.

In the first place, we can correctly speak of one person as
being *responsible to* another person or group. In this sense of
'responsibility' an employee is responsible to his/her employer,
and the Queen's ministers are responsible to Parliament. 'Responsible' here means the same as 'accountable', where
'accountable' means 'being obliged to explain and justify what
has been done'.

In the second place, we can speak of a person's being *responsible for* something, in the sense that it is his/her task or job or role to deal with it. This usage is often combined with the first, as when one says that a gardener is responsible *to* his employer *for* the proper upkeep of his garden, or that the Minister of Housing is responsible *to* Parliament *for* the state of the nation's housing. But we sometimes speak of a person's being responsible *for* something when there is no one to whom he/she may be said to be responsible. For example, we might say that adults are responsible for looking after their own health. What a person is responsible for in this sense may be called *responsibilities*. For example, we say, 'The care of your health is your own responsibility' or 'Your responsibilities as school gardener are to keep the garden looking attractive and to provide playing space for the children.'

Third, we speak of someone as being responsible and mean that he/she is reliable or conscientious or has a 'sense of responsibility'.

Fourth, a person can be responsible for something in the sense that he/she causes it to happen. This usage subdivides into (a) simply causing something to happen, and (b) causing something to happen where there can be implications of praise and blame. For example, if I am pushed and fall through a shop window I am responsible for the breakage simply in being a causal factor. In this sense, a blocked carburettor can be responsible for the breakdown of the car or poor weather for the bad harvest. But we also say, 'She was responsible for the muddle in the arrangements' and mean not only that she muddled them but also that she was blameworthy; or we say, 'She was responsible for the beautiful floral arrangements' and mean that she arranged the flowers in a praiseworthy manner. Notice that this sense of 'responsible for' is different from the second sense above. For, using being 'responsible for' in the earlier sense, we might say, 'You are responsible for the flower arrangements and yet have done nothing about them!'

Fifth, we speak of the 'age of responsibility' or say that 'responsibility was impaired'. To be responsible in this sense is to have the ability to make up one's own mind on what one wants or ought to do (to be autonomous) and to have the freedom to do it. All the other senses except simply causing something to happen presuppose that a person is already responsible in this last sense. In other words, they all presuppose that he/she is autonomous, for to be autonomous is to be individually responsible or accountable for one's behaviour. We shall call this view 'individualism'.

2. INDIVIDUAL RESPONSIBILITY AND HEALTH CARE

If individual responsibility or accountability is basic in that it underlies *responsibility to* somebody and *responsibilities for* something, it must also underlie the various kinds of responsibility found in health care contexts. Can there then in any sense at all be such a thing as collective or group or team responsibility in health care?

The answer would at first seem to be 'no', for if collectives are acting we cannot also say that individuals are acting, and if individuals are not acting we do not have morally responsible health care. But this argument is confused. If a voice at the end of the telephone says 'This is the Newton Health Centre' we do not imagine that the voice proceeds from anything other than an individual person (unless, of course, a telephone answering machine!). This suggests that there is a misleading disjunction between individual action and responsibility and collective action and responsibility, that it does not follow from the fact that a collective is acting that some individual person or persons are not also acting and responsible.

Why then would the individualist want to speak at all of 'collective' action and responsibility? One answer might be that it is convenient to do so − that it can be useful to use the idea of a collective to refer to the sum total of the actions and responsibilities of a group of associated individuals. For example, in medicine doctors are often part of a *group practice*. There are obvious advantages in group practices for doctors and patients in the provision of continuous patient care throughout the year or the sharing of expensive equipment. A group practice in this sense is a collective, but there is no incompatibility with the doctrine of individual moral responsibility. In terms of this first model of collective responsibility the actions of a collective, such as a group practice, are divisible into the actions of the individual doctors, who are each independently responsible for what they do. There is an analogy here with a dandelion, which consists of a number of flowers. Collective responsibility in this sense is the responsibility of aggregates.

Doctors also work in *teams* attached to health centres involving nurses, dentists, physiotherapists, social workers, and many other health care workers. Each of these health workers is individually responsible for his own contribution to a different aspect of health care, but in so far as they are part of one team there will be one individual who has overall responsibility. This is the collective responsibility of a hierarchy, and it is another sort of collective responsibility which is compatible with the first model to the extent that there is one person who has ultimate authority to take decisions. Aggregative and hierarchical responsibility together or separately might be thought to enable us to make sense of hospitals, health committees and all other apparent collectives in health care without at all forcing us to abandon or modify the strong doctrine of individual responsibility.

3. ROLES AND COLLECTIVE RESPONSIBILITY

However, there are serious limitations to this first simplistic model of individual responsibility in health care. Take first the basic idea of the practice of medicine, and let us grant that when a nurse or doctor acts, an individual acts. The important point which is obscured by this truism is that they are acting not *as individuals but as a nurse or as a doctor*, that is as an individual who has not only certain skills but also certain statutory and professional rights and duties. Similarly, a physiotherapist is acting *as a physiotherapist*, a dentist *as a dentist*, and so on.

We could approach this point in another way. The doctor aims at health and has the expertise relevant to promoting health, or to removing impediments to health. And the same is true for all the other health workers. It follows that these activities intimately bear on human good and harm. But we can now stress that in so far as the health care professional's activities bear intimately on human good and harm, the state will take an interest in them, and lay down broad conditions for qualifications and the running of health care professions. In other words, official health care activities are governed by legal statute. For example, there will be legislation laying down in general or specific terms the situations in which a patient has a legal right to medical care or to hospitalization. There may even be cases, perhaps of certain infectious or psychiatric disorders, where the doctor has a duty to commit the patient to care against his wishes. In the latter case, the authority by which a person may be compulsorily detained in a hospital obtains legally in Britain from an Act of Parliament. Indeed, the doctor, nurse, or social worker are specifically given protection in case of civil or criminal proceedings arising from the carrying out of any of these compulsory duties, provided they have not acted 'in bad faith or without reasonable care'. Whatever the details of legislation, it is clear that the bond which holds health care professional and patient together is at the least first a legal one.

The bond is constituted, second, by rather vaguer sets of rules, or even expectations, which health care workers and patients have of each other. There are many different facets to these. For example, a patient has the assurance that a doctor will not take advantage of him with respect to any information about his private life which emerges; and there will be no gossip about medical conditions or social predicaments. The medical profession is very strict about enforcing its own discipline on these matters. Reciprocally, a doctor would expect a patient to tell the truth and to try to carry out prescribed treatment. Social workers, for example, go as far as speaking of a 'contract' between themselves and their clients. These quasi-legal bonds, some of which are mentioned in codes of ethics, lie within the sphere of the 'ethical', as that term has been narrowly and traditionally understood in health care. (See introduction to Chapter 20.)

It is important that health care relationships should be constituted, at least partly, by these legal and quasi-legal institutional bonds, for at least the following reasons. First, because doctors, nurses, and all health and welfare workers, by the nature of their jobs, intervene in crucial ways in the lives of others. This is a serious matter and its consequences for a patient or client can be enormous. It is therefore in the interests of patients that there should be some sort of professional entitlement to intervene. In other words, if he is not simply to be a busybody, a doctor or social worker must have the *right to intervene*, and if he has the right to intervene, he must have duties and responsibilities; the concept of an institution encapsulates these ideas of rights, duties, and responsibilities.

A second reason is that doctors and other health care workers must ask about many intimate details of people's lives such as their marriages; and they also may conduct examinations of or have otherwise close contact with people's bodies. Questioning of this sort and intimate physical contact can create situations in which people can be exploited, or which could be embarrassing even to the professional workers themselves. The fact that it is an institutional bond which brings the doctor, nurse, or physiotherapist together with a patient provides *emotional insulation* for both parties in such situations. Moreover, since it is important that the professional worker should know these intimate details there must be some assurance that no untoward use be made of the information and that it will not be passed on as trivial gossip. But the idea of an institution entails that of rules, and the rules can, third, impose *confidentiality* on the professional workers and provide security for the patient.

Fourth, professionals are given a measure of *security* by virtue of the fact that they work inside an institutional framework. There are various aspects of this. For instance, it is good for all professions to have ways and means whereby new skills and knowledge can be shared and, in general, whereby members of a profession can support and encourage each other. Again, all health care professionals require legal or professional protection from exploitation, unfair criticism, or legal action against them by their patients. Reciprocally there must be some institutional mechanism whereby the professions can criticize themselves and look for ways of improving their services to the public. These then are some of the reasons for which a complex legal and institutional structure has grown up governing directly and indirectly the relationships between health and welfare workers and their patients.

There are various desirable and a few undesirable aspects to this, but the relevant point for our present purposes is that when the health worker appears to be acting as an individual he is also acting *as a representative* of his profession and to a lesser extent also of his state. In other words, the individual action of a doctor or other health worker expresses also the collective values of the relevant profession; individual responsibility becomes collective responsibility, since it is through the individual that the profession is represented. We might say that the individual health worker represents his profession in two senses. First, he is the ascriptive representative, in that the profession authorizes his actions, having sanctioned his training. Second, he represents the values of the profession in so far as he acts in terms of its ethics, and its ethics are all-pervasive in the actions and attitudes of the individual health worker.

But if the individual actions of the doctor or nurse are also the actions of collectives, what remains of the doctrine that individuals, and only they, can be held morally responsible for their actions? Here the concept of a social role is helpful as being a set of rights and duties to be analysed in terms of institutional concepts. An individual person is able to act not only in a private capacity but in that of a social role, and this concept, understood institutionally, enables us to do justice to the valid points in the collectivist's case, for it is not logically analysable in purely individualistic terms; its adequate specification must be in logically irreducible institutional terms. Yet the concept of social role, so understood, also enables us to do justice to the individualist's insistence that moral responsibility must remain with the individual person, for we can say that, if an individual consents to act in a role, he or she thereby becomes morally responsible for actions which are done in its name. In accepting the role, he identifies himself with the values of his profession and the rights and duties which go with the role. Moreover, by taking on the role we can say that the individuals are *authorized* by their professional associations to act in certain ways, depending on the function of the profession. Their authorization defines their professional values and their 'responsibilities to' and 'responsibilities for'.

This analysis enables us to improve on our first simplistic model of collective responsibility in health care. According to the first model the idea of collective responsibility was just a convenient fiction. The responsibility of the health team resolved itself into the individual responsibilities of the members of the team. Responsibility in the first sense is not *genuinely* collective. But we have tried to bring out in our second analysis that, in health care, responsibility must be genuinely collective. The reason for this is that in professional activities the individual nurse, doctor, dentist, and so on, is expressing the collective values of the respective profession.

These collective values change and develop over the years. Sometimes the changes are willingly brought about by the health care professions themselves, sometimes they are forced on the professions by the state or by public opinion. But always these collective values mould the roles and therefore influence the decisions and define the responsibilities of the members of the health care professions. The collective values of the professions are present in all the decisions of their individual members. That is why in all health care decisions there is genuine collective responsibility even when it is just an individual doctor, or nurse, or other who is deciding.

Before examining a third model of collective responsibility in health care we should note that although the collective values of professions mould the roles of health care there remains an enormous scope for individual initiative and the exercise of a whole range of individual skills and moral qualities in the *enactment* of the caring role. The difference between a good dentist or nurse and an indifferent one cannot lie in differences in roles, for the roles of each type of dentist, nurse or doctor will be the same. The difference lies in the personal qualities of skill, imagination, compassion, tact, patience, and so on which each brings to the role. The moral values expressed in all health care decisions are therefore partly the *collective* values of the profession expressed through its roles and partly the *individual* values of each person acting in his role.

4. HEALING AND COLLECTIVE RESPONSIBILITY

To develop a third model of collective responsibility in health care we shall turn from the roles to the skills and the aims of the health care professions.

Skills have an end, aim, or point which determines the nature of the skill. In the case of health care it is often said that the aim is to try to prevent or treat any illness or disease, malfunction, or injury which might interfere with human good. If we thus think of health care in terms of the removal of specific impairments or impediments we are likewise likely to think of the requisite skills as being in the possession of the individual professional who has responsibility for a given patient. The acceptability of this approach depends on the acceptability of the preceding account of the aim of health care. Is the account acceptable?

The weakness in it is that it adopts a narrow, even a negative, view of the aim of health care: it conceives the aim as being that of the removal of impediments to health. But there can also be a positive aspect to health. It is not merely the absence of discomfort and incapacity, but the positive feelings of a sense of fitness and energy, and a supple and well-tuned body − the condition in which someone is said to glow with health or be bursting with health. What may be seen as a luxury from the point of view of the negative aspect of health, such as the promotion of vigour in old age, is central from the point of view of the positive aspect. Medical concern with *contraception* can perhaps also be classified as the promotion of positive health, as being one element in physical pleasure and well-being. The aim of health care should therefore be seen not just negatively, as the attempt to free people from unwanted or abnormal conditions, but also positively. Indeed, we must go further and say that the aim of health care is not just that of promoting *health*, but should be even more broadly conceived as the promotion of 'wholeness'. Or, if it is thought that 'the promotion of wholeness' is too ambitious an aim, then we could employ the old-fashioned or religious-sounding noun 'healing', which covers more of the ground required for an adequate characterization of the aim of health care than our common modern word 'health'.

If we grant that the aim of health care including that of medicine should be thus broadly conceived as the promotion of the wholeness of a person, his 'healing', what follows about the nature of the skills and expertise required to promote it? The obvious implication is that the skills and expertise will be so varied that no one individual would be able to possess them all. Of course, the aim of the doctor could be re-stated in a way which would make it possible for the necessary skills to be in the possession of individual doctors at least in many cases. Thus, if we think in terms of our earlier-stated negative aim − the removing of impediments to normal functioning − then, in many cases at least, an individual doctor will have the skills necessary to promote that aim and, of course, a large part of medical work is concerned with just that. But if we think of the aim of medicine more positively, as the promotion of wholeness, of total well-being, than it is clear that what is required is a co-operative or collective exercise. Moreover, it will be a co-operative exercise of considerable breadth. To bring this out, consider the connections between health and welfare.

First of all, health is clearly one very important *part* of welfare in that it is reasonably wanted for its own sake and that possession of it is a necessary condition for pursuing very many other goals. For this reason part of the *social worker's job* will be to promote the health of his client: to encourage him to seek medical advice and to take it, and to help him cope with, for example, national health or other bureaucratic organizations.

This is not, of course, to say that the social worker may usurp the doctor's function of bringing his unique skill to bear on the patient's medical problems. But the social worker also has *responsibility* for the patient, which makes it quite reasonable that he should want to know what is going on medically. He may often also be the best person to *defend* the patient against the more narrowly conceived actions of the medical or nursing professions, where that is necessary: not where a *legal* defence is needed (for that he would have to call in another specialist!) but where firm presentations are needed by someone who has the confidence to address the doctor or nurse on equal terms as a fellow professional; about, say, over-persuasion by the doctor to undergo some experimental or controversial treatment, or about a refusal by the nursing staff to allow parents of young children to visit them in hospital.

We have said that the possession of health is a necessary condition for the pursuit of many other goals. The vital importance of this point will be clear when it is remembered how often a person becomes a 'social work case' because he is unable to hold down a job through chronic physical ill-health or alcoholism or mental illness; the immediate problem may be his lack of financial means, but the underlying cause of the problem is a *medical* one, even if the client thinks of himself as a social work rather than as a medical case. It is often for such medical reasons, too, that a person (for example, a neglectful parent or violent spouse) damages the interests of *others* to the extent that social workers become involved. In such cases the social worker needs to be able to consult the doctor on questions which are partly but not wholly medical: Has this man sufficiently recovered from his depression to be encouraged to look for a job? Is this woman likely to recover quickly from her mental illness and be able to look after her children again, or must long-term plans be made for them?

The second connection between health and welfare is of course the dependence of mental and physical health on other aspects of welfare, both material and non-material. To take an obvious example, an old person's health may be impaired because his house is damp, or has too many stairs, or because he cannot afford proper clothes, food or heating, or because he is not sufficiently able-bodied to look after himself. In all these situations, the expertise in specifying what is needed may be the doctor's, but the expertise in *getting* it, through statutory or voluntary services, is that of the social worker. The skill required to thread the maze of regulations and to persuade officialdom of the urgency of need can be considerable. There are also cases where the dependence of health on welfare is at a deeper level, as in those instances of psychiatric or physical illnesses which seem to be bound up with family or personal problems, and here the doctor may need social work help not only in alleviating the problem but also in understanding it.

It should emerge from these fairly obvious considerations that health and welfare are inextricably bound together and that the doctor and the social worker can each be − *must* each be − ancillary workers to the other, rather than mutually antagonistic, if these twin aims are to be achieved. The thrust of this line of argument will be towards breaking the idea that doctors, social workers, and other similar professionals ought to have their own separately identifiable aims of health or welfare. It seems preferable to minimize the differences in the specific aims of these professions and rather to see them all as 'caring' professions aiming at 'wholeness', and to have some interchange-ability of roles. Indeed, if we consider the importance in contemporary life of health education, of legislation to control pollution, and in general to maintain the environment it becomes evident that responsibility for 'wholeness' must be widely distributed.

We can draw the conclusion from this section of the argument that responsibility for health care must be collective in a third sense. In terms of the first (inadequate) model collective responsibility was completely analysable into individual responsibility. The second model was concerned with the institutional side of health care. It brought out the point that even if the health worker was acting as an individual he was also acting in a role as an authorized representative of a profession with the rights, duties, and values of the profession. This second model of collective responsibility we could think of as 'vertical'. The third model, by contrast, is horizontal, in the sense that responsibility for 'wholeness' (of which 'health' is a component) is shared by a wide variety of professions.

5. COMMUNITY RESPONSIBILITY

There is a fourth model of collective responsibility for health care, which is the most important of all. It can be introduced by a criticism which is often made of all the health care professions and has been given its most trenchant formulation by Ivan Illich.* The criticism is that health care workers and the whole context of health care have become what we might term 'over-professionalized'. The impression has been conveyed over several decades that an ordinary person cannot really manage his own health and welfare, and that for any of the ills of life there is an expert who will help him.

There are three connected aspects to this criticism. The first is what we might call the medicalization of ordinary experience. In other words, we have all been encouraged to think that every human anxiety, discomfort, or misery is a medical or related problem. Where in the past people might have thought that sleeplessness was something that you could treat yourself, that anxiety or grief were to be shared with a clergyman, a friend, or a neighbour, or that discomforts or miseries were to be put up with until they went away, we now turn to the doctor for a pill.

Going along with the medicalization of experience there is, secondly, the complementary belief that for every ailment there is an expert to help. Those in the health care business have not discouraged either of these beliefs and have warned of the dangers of not consulting the doctor in time, of not contacting welfare services, of not having regular checks on one's teeth, and so on.

The outcome of this takes us to the third and most important point for present purposes. The medicalization of ordinary experience plus the rise of the expert has had the result that people have lost confidence in their own abilities to take responsibility for their own health in particular and their own lives in general. Ordinary people have come to feel that they do

*See Bibliography.

not have the expertise needed to help with family or similar difficulties. As a consequence many people have lost the feeling that there is a moral need to have any concern for one's neighbour; 'they' can now be relied on to do everything.

The care for all these ills is the same; health care workers must abandon their professional isolation and begin to work *through* the community rather than *on* it. To be fair, there are many signs that this has begun to happen. For example, there is greater stress than there used to be on *community* medicine and dentistry, which are educative and preventive, trying to get people to look after their own health or teeth as far as they can. The media have been encouraged by the health care professions and governments to carry programmes on the dangers of smoking and the importance of a proper diet. Again, community social workers aim to get people to help each other, rather than doing the helping themselves *de haut en bas*. There has in fact been a growth in recent years of self-help groups − from the familiar 'Alcoholics Anonymous' groups to the many types of parents' groups concerned with education, bereavement and every sort of serious childhood disease. The growth of such self-help movements should be encouraged and informed by those in professional health care.

6. CONCLUSION

We can now make explicit the fourth and most important model of collective responsibility in health care. For adequate health care, for wholeness, we require not just that we should be served by authorized representatives with the rights, duties, skills, and values of the health care professions (our second sense of collective responsibility), not just that these representatives should co-operate in teams for our total, positive health (our third sense); for wholeness we require that we should all see ourselves as members of a collectively responsible society (our fourth sense). In other words, the members of the health care professions must be assisted by our own striving to become (in the words of St Paul) 'members one of another'. This idea of a collectively responsible society, of a public or community good or welfare (as distinct from an aggregate of individual goods), is presupposed by the medical, nursing, and social services specialty of public health. (See Chapter 15.)

Chapter 7

MORAL CONFLICT AND MORAL DEFICIENCY

In considering the responsibilities of professional workers for health care we noted that the personal moral qualities of an individual — his/her role-enactment or sense of responsibility — can enhance the performance of official duties or responsibilities. But the personal moral outlook of a professional worker does not always blend harmoniously with the performance of official duties. There are two types of cases where there might be a lack of blending.

In the first type the professional is instructed by a senior to carry out or assist with some treatment of which he or she disapproves in moral terms. For example, it is well-known that some nurses disapprove of abortions, and assisting with one would be morally repugnant to those so minded. Again, some mental nurses disapprove of electroconvulsive therapy and would feel morally compromised if expected to assist. In another area of medicine, moral conflicts can arise over instructions to resuscitate certain patients, or over the question whether certain patients should not be told the truth about their conditions. It is typical of this first type of case that those who are in conflict with their seniors may hold strongly the view that their seniors are morally wrong in what they are advocating and try to persuade them to change their minds.

In the second type of case the doctor, nurse, or social worker in some way falls short of the moral quality required for the performance of their jobs, for an adequate role-enactment. This kind of case has many subdivisions. For example, it is well-known that depression among dentists, doctors, and other health care workers does sometimes lead to problems of alcoholism or drug abuse. The case of the 'sick doctor' is familiar in medical literature. Deficiencies of this kind are clearly going to affect professional practice. Another kind of moral deficiency can be seen where a doctor, for example, has a financial motive for urging a certain kind of treatment, perhaps a private clinic. Here his private interests may be adversely affecting his professional life. Most commonly there are instances where there is an inadequacy in the quality of performance of the official duties, in the role-enactment. Serious cases of this come under the heading of negligence and as such are within the jurisdiction of the law. However, we are also concerned with an overlapping set of cases which do not on the whole fall within the scope of the law but which nevertheless constitute a kind of moral negligence, a falling short of a standard of conduct which might reasonably be expected of a profession. This is the sort of deficiency which professional colleagues notice and worry about. Let us call this type of failing 'moral deficiency' to distinguish it from the first type, which we shall call 'moral conflict'.

1. MORAL CONFLICT

In cases of moral conflict it is helpful to distinguish three points of view; that of the person carrying out the treatment, that of the profession or senior representative of it, and that of the patient. One approach might be that, in cases of conflict between these three perspectives, the doctor or nurse should simply ignore his or her own attitude and carry out treatment or procedures according to the consensus prevailing in the profession at any given period. In other words, if in doubt or conflict, do what the others in one's peer group are doing. There is merit in this proposal, in that one needs good reason to be out of step with what others in the same line of business are doing, especially since, as we have said, a doctor or nurse is a representative of a profession. But, on the other hand, it never follows that because others are in fact doing something one ought to be doing it, too; perhaps they have never much thought about it and are in the wrong.

A second approach is to urge that what ought to have priority is the patient's perspective, that we ought to do what the patient wants. In childbirth, for example, we hear of the mother-to-be arriving with a 'shopping list' of her requirements, and no doubt this demand can be generalized and lead to the conclusion that the doctor or nurse should simply be carrying out the patient's wishes. This is a strong version of a doctrine of patients' rights or patients' autonomy.

In reply to this we must first note, as we have maintained in Chapter 2, that patients do not always know what they want, and frequently appeal to the professional to decide for them. This need not be an irrational abdication of responsibility on the part of the patient, for the patient may reasonably judge that a doctor or nurse will have much more experience of a treatment or procedure and is therefore in a better position to decide. Second, we must remember that doctors and nurses also have rights to autonomy, and a woman's right to choose entails that someone in the profession has a duty to implement the right. But if the duty is to fall on a doctor or nurse then they are entitled to decide whether or not they accept what is proposed as a duty.

Moreover, there can be important resource implications for doctors, nurses, and nowadays managers, if they defer against their better judgements to the demands of individual patients or relatives. The medical and managerial responsibility is to a given population of patients, to manage a limited budget in a fair and efficient manner. In other words, justice and utility are ethical principles which must temper the full implementation of the demands of some individual patients.

The criticisms of the first two approaches seem to bring us back to the doctrine of the absolute moral responsibility of the individual doctor or nurse for what he or she does. This, as we have suggested, seems to be an implication of the moral autonomy of the doctor or nurse. What then should happen if there is a conflict of moral views? It might seem that, faced with an instruction with which he morally disagrees, the professional with a high sense of moral responsibility ought to resign. Now no doubt there are important issues of the kind that require resignation rather than compliance, but for most matters this is much too drastic a solution and, if we are thinking of resignation from a job rather than just a committee, it is also unrealistic. What then is the solution, the middle way between ignoring one's own moral attitude and resigning if one disagrees?

The first point in the moderate solution is that one can try to anticipate a difficult situation and prevent it arising. For example, a nurse might anticipate that she will be expected to take part in some policy of concealing the truth from a patient. She should raise the matter with a senior nurse before she is actually instructed to do so, for most people are willing to listen to arguments. None the less, it takes tact and courage to indicate one's doubts or disagreements. That is one reason why we earlier stressed the importance for all health care workers of developing certain qualities of character in themselves. Of course, to have the courage and tact to raise one's moral problems with senior persons does not mean that they will always change their minds and agree.

This takes us to the second point. In Chapter 4 we stressed that respecting persons means that one must recognize that they may have moral values which differ from one's own. Moral argument must therefore be conducted in an open way without entrenched positions, without assuming at the onset that one must always be right. Sometimes, if we approach moral argument in the right spirit, the person whose mind we set out to change may change our own mind! Or, what is perhaps more common, we come to have a better understanding of another point of view even if we still disagree with it. In a practical profession, however, there must always in the end be decisions as to what ought to be done, and what a senior professional decides ought to be done may not be what one thinks oneself to be the right course of action. Here it is important to draw a distinction between compromising one's conscience for expediency, a quiet life or a good reference for one's next job, and a conscientious compromise (see pp. 17–18). In other words, a certain decision may not be the one which ideally we should have reached ourselves, but granted the complexities of a real situation, the patient's views, the views of our professional peers, the views of our seniors, we should generally go along with what in our own opinion may not be ideal.

To say this is not to modify the doctrine of the moral autonomy of the individual but simply to say that the moral life is hard! Indeed, it may be said that the moral agent is never responsible for the total content of an action. The situation in which he finds himself, whether in public, professional, or private life, is never one of which he is the sole creator, since he is born into an environment not of his making; his moral actions, being reactions to his situation, are necessarily affected by it.

Our solutions (or rather our suggestions, for there are no solutions) to the problems of moral conflict in professional life, then, are to anticipate and prevent where possible, and to modify and compromise where that is not possible. No doubt, in extreme situations, the health care professional should refuse to compromise (Nazi doctors, Soviet psychiatrists, etc.).

2. MORAL DEFICIENCY

What we are concerned with under this heading is not mainly the failure in the performance of duties by a professional person. Failure in the performance of duties is usually a matter of negligence, although of course it is also moral failure of a serious kind. We shall here be concerned with less serious but more pervasive moral failures which are not caught in the legal net. Most often these are failures or inadequacies in the *manner* in which patients are treated, rather than in the substance of their treatment; they are inadequacies in what in our previous chapter we have called the role-enactment. In particular these in-adequacies are most often shown in the *attitude* which a health care worker may have to a patient or client, or in their relationships with one another.

One type of attitude to which health care workers are prone is that of paternalism. We are not here thinking of a failure in applying legal requirements of informed consent to treatment, but rather of a more subtle form of the same; namely, the failure to explain to a patient what is happening, why certain activities are taking place and what effects are to be expected. Instead of doing these things as appropriate the paternalistic professional will smile benignly and say 'Don't you worry, everything is going fine'. This kind of attitude is patronizing and hurtful, because it conveys that the patient is not capable of understanding anything, or that the patient is too unimportant to be worth the trouble of an explanation. It must be remembered also that patients are in a vulnerable position, because the professional is at home in the care setting and has power over the patient or client. The power of the professional can be conveyed in all sorts of ways, as for example by standing over the patient, or speaking about him to others in his presence. This is irresponsible behaviour in that it shows a lack of respect for the autonomy or dignity of the person who happens to be a particular client. (See Chapter 11, section 4.)

A second form of this morally irresponsible attitude is shown when a professional implies that the patient's wants, fears, and anxieties are all to be construed as causally produced by the illness or related to psychological factors, and therefore to be treated as symptoms rather than as expressions of genuine purposes or rational desires. For example, a doctor, nurse, or social worker might say 'You will see things differently when you are well again'. Or a doctor might say to a nurse about a patient, 'Don't worry about that patient's complaints. He's angry because that's one of the stages which dying patients go through.' In both cases the effect is to undercut the reasons which the patient himself would give for his actions or thoughts, and replace them by mechanisms on which the doctor, nurse, or social workers would claim to be an expert. The motivation for doing this may be, as we said in Chapter 5, the wish to avoid genuine encounters with people.

But just as often health care professionals have no such ulterior motive and may simply believe that they know more about what the patient does, thinks, or feels than the patient himself. In either case, the implication is that the patient is not to be regarded as an autonomous being who acts in pursuance of his own purposes and has genuine questions to ask.

Doctors and nurses are tempted into the first form of this inappropriate attitude by their superior knowledge and power, which make for paternalism; and they are tempted into the second by the carry-over into the doctor – or nurse–patient relationship of inappropriate causal models found in some social sciences. (See Chapter 8, section 1.)

All this may seem unreasonable to some doctors and nurses. After all, they will say, we are dealing all the time with people who on any reckoning are governed to a more than average extent by non-rational factors. Even if we leave aside the cases of mental illness, doctors and nurses are often dealing with people whose rationality is impaired by physical illness or pain, or who are affected by drugs. We have discussed this in Chapter 5. It is therefore not morally irresponsible to adopt the causal attitudes derived from the social sciences to patients.

There is much truth in this objection, as we saw earlier on, but two points must be borne in mind in mitigation of it. The first is that there is always a temptation, which must be guarded against, to extend this attitude beyond those patients, and those aspects of patients, which would justify it. The temptation exists because adopting a detached casual attitude to patients is often an easier option than taking them seriously. The second is that it may be therapeutic to express a genuine respect for a patient's autonomy even in cases which may not fully justify it. The policy of treating people as rational unless proved otherwise may have the effect of fostering rationality, which is not an all-or-nothing matter.

A third area in which a professional's attitude may sometimes be defective is in the exercise of what we have called compassion. In Chapter 4 we included the attitude of compassion as an important ingredient in respect, but the showing of compassion in a busy daily routine may not be easy. For example, a doctor who in abstract terms would see himself as devoted to the relief of suffering may still speak brusquely or insensitively to a patient. What is morally required is a kind of steady maintenance of the awareness that a patient has a capacity to suffer. Such an attitude is, of course, required of all of us, but is especially vital to the health care worker and is also more likely to be eroded by familiarity with suffering.

A fourth area in which the attitude or manner of a health care professional may be praiseworthy or blameworthy is in respect of the personal interest he or she takes in the human being who happens to be the patient. This quality is especially important to the nurse, the general practitioner, or the social worker, who are perhaps in more constant contact with a patient than the average hospital doctor or school dentist, but it is important also to all carers. The conditions for a personal friendship do not generally hold in the patient—professional relationship; what most patients want and need is better described as 'befriending'. As we have already stressed there is always a temptation to avoid personal encounters by seeing patients just as patients, rather than as people who happen to be ill. Personal encounters can be avoided, as we have seen, by paternalism or by trying to understand people in terms of causal mechanisms, but they can also be avoided by hiding behind 'professionalism' and the formality which goes with it. Indeed, some accounts of professional—patient relationships actually discourage the display of anything 'personal' in relationships with patients. But even a brief indication on the part of the nurse or doctor that they are human beings as well as professional carers may be welcomed by a patient: or a personal enquiry about the patient's life outside the consulting room or hospital may transform the relationship, or rather, it may put it in true perspective as one kind of a truly human relationship.

In thinking about moral deficiency in health care one tends to think of the inadequacy as located in the relationship between health care professional and patient, but problems can also arise in professional jealousies between different health care professions, and in the training of professionals.

The first of these types of problem arises because of the dual nature of professions. Professions are generally portrayed by their members as existing for the benefit of their patients or clients, by providing services and supervising and authorizing training programmes. In terms of this approach the criteria for the success of a profession, or a member of it, should derive from this outward-looking aim. But professions are also inward-looking, concerned with holding on to monopolies of their services in the face of rivalry from other groups, with improving their salaries and status at the expense of other groups and so on. When this aspect of professional life is dominant than rivalries will break out. For example, there are rivalries between barristers and solicitors, especially about appearances in courts, and in health care the traditional dominance of doctors is being challenged by nurses; and some aspects of traditional nursing roles, such as helping patients to walk again after operations, have been taken over by other professionals. Such rivalries are inevitable as professions change and develop but it can be hypocritical to pretend that the aim of the professional is always improved patient care.

A less commonly noted aspect of the tensions which arise between the needs of the profession and the needs of individual patients can be called the trainee's dilemma.* This dilemma can be introduced by drawing attention to an implicit contradiction between two clauses in the World Medical Association Declaration of Geneva (see p. 270). The first clause states that the physician will pledge himself to the service of humanity, whereas the third clause states that the health of the patient is the first consideration. Now the service of humanity clearly requires that there should be a constant supply of health care professionals, and that implies that trainees must practise their skills on patients, no doubt under supervision. But the best interests of the patient are served by treatment administered by the trained expert rather than the novice. This dilemma becomes acute in certain kinds of surgery -say ophthalmic surgery − where at crucial stages in an operation there cannot be dual control. In other words, the trainee is on his own in an irreversible way − good experience for him, but for the patient?

The solution to this dilemma, as far as morality is concerned, is to invoke the distinction stated in Chapter 1 between compromising our consciences and conscientious compromises. The

*See Newton, Michael J. (1986). Moral dilemmas in surgical training. *Journal of Medical Ethics*, **12**, 4.

trainee and his teacher must compromise, in that the 'service of humanity', which requires a constant supply of trained professionals, must be balanced against the duty of providing the best possible treatment for a given patient. But the compromise must be conscientious in that the trainee must have a sincere and realistic self-appraisal of his capabilities. Sometimes one hears a distinguished but youthful musician asked whether he plans to play a certain concerto. He may reply that he is not ready for it yet. He does not mean that he cannot play the notes, but rather that he feels that he does not yet have the artistic maturity to do justice to the work. This is not so much modesty as a realistic self-appraisal. In a similar way the trainee, encouraged by a teacher, must develop a realistic self-appraisal. This is as valid for the student nurse as for the moderately experienced surgeon, and it is an important part of having a sense of responsibility. To go ahead with an operation simply to give oneself some practice is a serious kind of moral deficiency.

A final, and controversial, point about moral deficiencies in the enactment of professional roles concerns the private life of the professional. It is well known that doctors may be severely disciplined for sexual relationships with their patients, even if these are part of private rather than professional life. But can a nurse or doctor play a convincing part in health education (which we regard as an important part of their role) and also smoke or over-eat or over-drink themselves? Magistrates or sheriffs have had to resign their professional posts because of convictions for drunken driving − presumably because in sentencing others for the same offence they would lack credibility. Do health care workers not in a similar way lack credibility if in their private lives their habits are at odds with the professed values of their callings? Perhaps for the health care professional his home cannot be his castle.

3. CONCLUSION

We have seen that a health care worker's personal moral qualities may pull away from what is required by the professional role.

This can occur either when someone disagrees with what may be required in a professional capacity, or when there are some personal moral inadequacies getting in the way of the best professional performance. In both types of case − moral conflict and moral deficiency − the ideal is the achievement of moral unity in life, the sincerity and realistic self-appraisal which come from being a good person who happens to be a nurse, doctor, dentist, social worker, or other health care worker.

Chapter 8

ALTERNATIVE VIEWS
OF HUMAN NATURE

We have analysed health care problems in terms of a moral philosophy which has 'respect for persons' as its basic principle, and in Part 2 we shall illustrate this principle in detailed health care examples. It would be misleading to suggest however that this is the only way of looking at health care problems. Indeed, we have made only a modest claim in Part 1, that we are providing a *model* of human nature and morality — a simplified way of looking at it. Within the complex and inconsistent moral views to be found in the health care professions there are many other elements to which we have not so far referred. In an attempt to make partial redress we shall refer to some other implicit or explicit systems of value which influence the practice of health care.*

1. THE BIOMEDICAL MODEL

To set the scene for these alternative views we shall begin by outlining the system of value which is often thought to be implicit in health care. This is called 'the biomedical model' of human nature and it is said to be derived from the scientific base of

*The idea of this chapter originated in CCETSW Paper 13 (1976). See Bibliography.

health care. It is a mechanistic view of human nature. According to this view (of which the modern source is Thomas Hobbes in the seventeenth century) human nature is simply matter in motion, and human thought and action can all ultimately be explained in terms of the laws of physics and chemistry. A powerful twentieth-century form of this view is to be found in behavioural psychology. Influenced originally by the work of Pavlov on conditioned responses, behavioural psychologists have developed complicated theories based on concepts such as 'drive' which are intended to be seen in some way as bridging the gap between purposive models of human behaviour and purely physiological models. All such theories base their methods on traditional science and stress their empirical scientific approach. In doing so they adopt the philosophy or paradigm of the sciences on which they have modelled themselves and thus implicitly take up a philosophical position about human beings; one, moreover, which has implications for the nature of all health care intervention.

One implication is this. If human beings are in the end complex conditioned response mechanisms then the appropriate way to treat them is by means of sophisticated systems of rewards and punishments, and effort spent on trying to get them to *understand* their situation is irrelevant to the model used. The term 'patient' will literally be the appropriate one, for they will be seen as passive, to be worked upon causally. The appropriate moral attitude will be paternalism. It is most unfortunate that the idea is widespread that this is the 'medical model' of human nature, for it is a model that ignores the creative energies of human beings and their abilities to assist in their own healing process.

One motivation for the adoption of this view of human nature by the health care professions is the belief that it is 'scientific' and therefore value-free. But this is an illusion. Certainly, bodily or mental states may be changed using science-based techniques, but the *direction* of therapy is value determined, for it is decided by the health care worker in accordance with some set of beliefs, which may be unspecified, or even unacknowledged, about right, good, or appropriate behaviour. Thus, the most scientific techniques incorporate values in the philosophy they wittingly or unwittingly adopt in developing their methods as well as in the uses to which they are later put. Our point, however, is that this mechanistic view is by no means required for the practice of health care and is by no means the most satisfactory way of looking at human nature. Despite the term 'biomedical model' it is not the model adopted in this book.

2. THE PSYCHOANALYTICAL MODEL

A second view of human nature which has direct implications for health care is psychoanalytic theory. The system would not appear to carry the same value difficulty because its aim is to encourage insight and therefore increase freedom of choice in the patient. But whereas this is the general aim of the theory, experience has shown that it can be used manipulatively, and under those circumstances carries the same value problems as mechanistic approaches.

However that may be, it is certainly true that psychoanalysis and the various developments of dynamic psychology which have stemmed from it have profoundly influenced our contemporary conception of human nature. It represents an important approach to the development of personality and character and provides a framework for understanding current behaviour in the light of past experience. It emphasizes self-knowledge and the complexity of human interaction. The stress placed on unconscious mental processes as powerfully affecting the springs of human action has had wide repercussions and has become part of the intellectual climate of our times.

Freud's original interest was in the treatment of patients suffering from neurotic symptoms. In listening to their descriptions of their symptoms he observed repeated patterns or themes which took the form of erotic or aggressive fantasies. These themes appeared to be repetitions of childhood fantasies stemming from early relationships. If these were pointed out to patients and if it was shown how they repeated these in present-day relationships, particularly with the analyst (the concept of 'transference') patients displayed anxiety and surprise which were followed gradually by a change, at least in symptom patterns. The patients' reactions of surprise and their lack of awareness that their symptoms had the same form as their childhood fantasy or of their own adult erotic or aggressive wishes suggested some active mental agency keeping such themes from conscious experience (mechanisms of defence).

Freud then noted the similarity of many everyday acts to neurotic symptoms and extended his propositions more generally to human behaviour and experience. Thus, he postulated that an important part of mental life is unconscious; some consciously experienced acts are symbolic representations of unconscious activity. The unconscious themes seem to be insistent and repetitive and mental life can thus be conceived as driven by unconscious forces.

Conflict could exist between conscious and unconscious forces and also between conflicting urges. Freud used these ideas, along with others about the irrational guilt which he observed in patients, in his conception of the psychic structure: this was composed of the *id*, which is the mental representation of body urge, the *ego*, which is the representation of external reality, and the *super-ego*, the representation of organized self-scrutiny which gives rise to guilt. The *ego* was seen as the agency which assimilates various conflicting tendencies or forces.

Following Freud, and based on his work, a whole body of psychodynamic theory was developed. For example, fantasies of young children were studied. Again, other psychoanalysts developed the idea of projection − the tendency (for defence purposes) for people to endow others with attributes which they do not wish to experience about themselves. Other psycho-analysts stressed the importance of projection by large groups on to others (nationalism, prejudice, racism, etc.) and by small groups like the family. More generally, stress has been placed on the importance of the early environment in understanding people: the child's relations with parents, patterns of relating within families, the social (national, tribal) context of families. It was held that any study of individuals was incomplete unless it considered them in their group settings. In this way, psychodynamic theory came to be incorporated in social psychology. It continues to have a great impact on the study and treatment of psychosomatic and psychological illness, and most health care work is to some extent influenced by it.

3. EXISTENTIALISM

Very different from the first and second of these views of man is that of the Existentialist. Existentialism arose as a protest against the view that man has a fixed nature or essence. The main tradition of moral thinking from Plato (in religious and secular form) asserted in a variety of ways that man has a nature which can be realized in his actions to the extent that they embody or conform to objective values − that there is truth or falsity in morality as in the world of fact. The Existentialists from Kierkegaard to Sartre reject this model of man. For them man has no fixed nature; he creates himself in his choices. The emphasis is on human freedom to choose. Indeed, the nearest Existentialist analogue to the traditional idea of moral wrong-doing is the failure to exercise one's freedom in authentic choice and the seeing of oneself as determined by circumstance, environment, or physical make-up.

Existentialism has influenced some schools of psychiatry and social work because it has seemed to them to offer practical guidance in a way in which much traditional academic philosophy does not. It stresses human freedom and choice and brings home to health care workers the marked extent to which their clients lack these features, assumed to be basic rights of man. One might say that whereas traditional academic philosophers have *discussed* the nature of human freedom the Existentialists have urged their followers to *experience* freedom and to *practise* it. The philosophy of mechanism and that of psychoanalysis can be seen as arising directly out of the scientific aspects of health care, while the school of existentialist psychiatry can be seen as a reaction to the manipulative and deterministic assumptions of science-based health care.

4. ZEN BUDDHISM

A fourth philosophy of human nature with its own distinctive values which are relevant to health care is that of Zen Buddhism. In particular, Zen Buddhism appeals to those who are attracted to holistic medicine and other forms of 'alternative medicine'. Some of the ideas have influenced the many millions of people in Western civilization who turn in their despair from their own destructive culture to Eastern ideas in the hope of finding salvation. Zen is not a philosophy or a psychology, in that it is not a system founded on logic or analysis and it has no structure. It is not a religion; it has no god, no dogma, no ideas of soul or immortality. The East does not care so much for details as the West and tends more to a comprehensive and intuitive grasp of the whole which is foreign to Western patterns of thought. Zen is an ultimate expression of this.

Zen basically is about insight; insight into the real nature of self. It is difficult to develop those ideas in a treatise such as ours because Zen baffles language. While some writings do exist, these came after the development of Zen and act as a rationale. Zen is experience − personal and individual − which is not readily expressed and, indeed, one of its main points is that we are too much slaves to words. It deals with facts and not with their representations; where words cease to correspond with facts then it leaves words and deal with facts. In similar fashion it goes beyond logic and common sense and aims to show that these ways of looking at things are not final.

The central perception of Zen is 'satori' − which may be translated as 'enlightenment'. Enlightenment is usually achieved only after long years of disciplined training during which time the mind is cleared of conscious suppositions (or assumptions). The impediments of consciousness, conventional habit patterns, logic and intellect, accepted understanding, etc., are broken through. Old groundwork is upset and reconstructed on an entirely new basis and when this is achieved there is a sudden flashing into consciousness of a new truth. This is satori.

Satori cannot be borrowed. It must grow out of the self. There is a strong insistence on inner spiritual experience, and personal experience is set above authority or objective revelation. In Zen there is therefore a strong element of apparent iconoclasm which is particularly evident in the sayings of many of the Zen masters.

Zen deals with steps in the development of consciousness in a way not readily acceptable to Western thought. There is a difference between consciousness of the existence of an object (an easily grasped concept in Western thought) and the development of consciousness of an object (an idea more easily grasped in the East). It is not that something different is seen but that the same thing is seen differently.

One important consequence of the Western interest in the Eastern religion has been the development of meditation and systems of exercise intended to assist in controlling the body so as to free the spirit from its interference. This technique is known as 'yoga' or the process of becoming yoked to the Absolute. Clearly, techniques of this kind are of great importance to health care and can be used even by those who do not attempt to understand the philosophy out of which the technique has emerged.

Existentialism and Zen Buddhism, and to some extent psychoanalytic theory, all represent views of man different from the mechanistic view arising out of modern science. They are widely different in their origins and general approach, but they have this in common that they resist the idea that the essential spirit of human beings can be caught in any slogan.

5. MARXISM

A fifth view of man and his condition is provided by Marxist theory. The Marxist view of man stresses the importance of man as a social animal defined by his social relationships. The distinctive feature of human nature is 'consciousness' which for the Marxist is a social product. Human consciousness develops through history so that historical knowledge is self-knowledge. Marxist theory stresses the importance of action and production in understanding human nature and criticizes the method of defining man in terms of his artefacts, whether these be material products or abstract concepts (for example, money or ideas).

This introduces the concept of 'alienation' which is fundamental to Marxist thinking. Man, by attributing independent existence and power to the products of his own mind or labour, is alienated from himself. These reified abstractions (e.g. religion, the state, capital) deprive men of their opportunities to perceive their true state and they are therefore trapped in false consciousness.

The Marxist depicts the development of history through class struggle as the development of man's consciousness. In our present society the bourgeois intellectual is seen as being in a particular dilemma in that he is engaged in a self-defeating task. He struggles to make his world comprehensible and in so doing unwittingly lays bare the contradictions in capitalist society, a society which must eventually collapse because it is organized in the interests of the minority.

The ideas and values which we hold and claim to be universal are seen as products of a minority but dominant group and serve to preserve its position. The central problem for contemporary man is his separation into subject and object. The structure of society prevents men from having a complete understanding of their predicament, and human potential is limited by compart-mentalizing and specialization. Men may act technically, as tools of production, or ethically. When they act ethically they retreat into privacy and emphasize individualism. The Marxist would agree with the Christian that the human predicament cannot be put right by individual effort, or indeed by what is usually meant by state intervention. He sees the only hope as lying in revolution in which the dominant classes in society will be overthrown along with the economic structure which made them dominant, and a new classless society will thereby emerge.

6. THE JUDAEO-CHRISTIAN TRADITION AND ISLAM

The Judaeo-Christian tradition and Islam have many points in common. We shall discuss Judaism and Christianity together, and say a little more about Islam since it is less familiar to Western readers although important for understanding the beliefs of an immigrant population. The Judaeo-Christian tradition is like Marxism to the extent that it is critical of existing social structures, but it is more ambiguous about the means of salvation. One strand in it is clearly world-rejecting, seeing the kingdom of heaven as something within the individual. It follows from this that the faith has nothing to say on the condition of the inner city, or nuclear disarmament. Another strand preaches a social gospel, as is illustrated in nineteenth-century evangelical movements, or in contemporary 'worker-priest' movements in Latin America. But while different emphases may be found within different strands, basically the Judaeo-Christian places primary emphasis on man's relationship with God and holds that relationship to be his goal and happiness; his responsibility to and relationship with his fellow man derive from it. Created in his image by God, man has a capacity for choice, and in exercising it makes a bid for independence and self-sufficiency. This ineradicable tendency to choose his own ends rather than discover God's purpose is called 'sin' and brought about physical death and a severance of the relationship between man and God. God takes the initiative in re-establishing the relationship, first through law and then, specifically for the Christian, through redemption. Christian teaching includes belief in both the immortality of the soul, and the resurrection of the body. Although man is capable of much good, his attempts to regain control over the world, his own nature, and his social relationships can never be completely successful through his own efforts; peace will ultimately be restored only through the re-establishment of God's rule on earth.

Central to Christian belief is the doctrine of the Incarnation: by becoming man, Christ revealed both the nature of God and the nature of man when he is in harmony with God. The essence of that nature is love. His death is the supreme expression of that love as his resurrection is of the ultimate triumph of good over evil and his followers are similarly enjoined to demonstrate love. Man's love of, and need for, his fellows are expressions of the divine love and God's own wish for relationship. It is in a community, both in the Church and in his secular life, that the Christian can best experience and express the love of God.

Different Judaeo-Christian traditions lay different emphases on the sinful nature of unredeemed man or on his essential goodness and perfectibility, and some give more place to individual and some to collective and racial experience. Some stress the righteousness and some the mercy of God; some attach more importance than others to the Church and its ordinances. All, however, see the ultimate hope of mankind in his re-established relationship with God, though some would see this as essentially expressed in his harmonious relationships with his fellow men.

The founder of Islam was Mohammed, an Arab who was born around AD 570. He made no claim to divinity himself and was more like an Old Testament prophet, such as Ezekiel, than like Jesus. Islam is the worship of Allah and submission to Allah. Mohammed, though inspired by Allah, is regarded as himself liable to error and even sin. It is therefore wrong to call the adherents of Islam 'Mohammedans'.

Mohammed taught that there is one God who has absolute and transcendent power. Allah, the mighty One, is separated from his creatures by an unbridgeable gulf and the whole duty of human beings is Islam (or submission). The follower of Islam is a Moslem, or a submissive one. The will of Allah is all-important, but completely arbitrary. But Moslems will point out that two of the many names of Allah are 'the compassionate' and 'the merciful'. On the other hand, it is clear from the historical development of Moslem doctrine that it lends itself to rigid fundamentalism and the fanaticism which accompanies fundamentalism. The ideal believer is personified submission.

The sacred book of Islam is the 'Koran', which means 'that which is uttered or recited'. It contains the revelations of Mohammed, which he received when he was inspired. Many of them are reminiscent of Christian moral teachings. For example:

The best and most beautiful of my creations is a compassionate man who gives alms. If he does so with his right hand and hides it from his left, he is more powerful than all things.

or

Anything that will bring a smile on the face of others is a good deed, and is the love of one's neighbours.

Sayings of this sort are clearly ideals for health care.

One reason for the development of Islam is the simplicity of the devotional exercises. These are:

> The recital of the creed 'There is no Deity but Allah, and Mohammed is his prophet'.
> The recital of daily prayers, accompanied by ablutions.
> Fasting, especially during the lunar month of Ramadan.
> Almsgiving.
> Pilgrimage to Mecca.
> Holy War.

From the health care point of view it is important to note that the consumption of pork and alcohol is utterly rejected, and sexual mores differ from Western ones.

7. COMPARISON AND IMPLICATIONS

These accounts of different theories of human nature are greatly over-simplified, but may serve to indicate some of the forms of thought which health care workers will encounter. They clearly differ in various ways from the moral philosophy of 'healthy respect' outlined so far in Part 1. We shall conclude this chapter by making some comparisons.

The philosophy dominant in health care might be called the 'liberal/Kantian' view because, as we have seen, it combines elements from the moral philosophy of Kant with that of J. S. Mill and other liberal thinkers. We have stressed that two human capacities, summed up in the word 'autonomy', are emphasized in this viewpoint: self-determination and self-government. The Jew, Christian, Moslem, Zen Buddhist, or the Marxist are not, of course, committed to denying that human beings have those capacities, but rather that they see other features of human beings and their situation as being the important ones, or the relevant ones. For example, the liberal view of human nature differs from the Christian in that it does not depict human nature as fundamentally in error but rather as a mixture of self-interested desires and benevolent desires, and hence more hope of improvement is held out by the liberal. The Moslem will see the good man as one who is not self-governing, but who submits his will to that of Allah. Again, the liberal will differ from the Marxist in that he will believe that social improvements can be brought about by co-operation with the state. In particular, he will stress the importance of education in bringing about social progress, and hope to see the steady improvement of the human condition as the state and voluntary organizations together lead to the gradual eradication of human ills.

Zen Buddhists hold that man's real nature is good but that the way to perceiving this is long and arduous. For them social improvements lie principally in the ability of individuals to reach their true nature. No system will work while it is operated by people caught up in their cravings for sex, prestige, status, material possessions, etc. The more they strive to achieve these apparent needs the further from a solution they must be. Conversely, any system generated by those who have attained satori would be humane.

The Christian, Moslem, Zen Buddhist, the liberal, and the psychoanalyst will each tend to be concerned with the individual, whereas the Marxist will be more interested in the social dimension of human ills. The Jew, Christian, and the liberal will regard it as worth while to argue with bureaucrats in order to try to persuade them to alter legislation, redistribute resources, etc., in what each regards as a more just way. The Marxist will tend to regard such efforts as futile because he will see institutional authorities as being essentially hostile to such improvements.

Another important point of comparison is the attitude to women encouraged by these different views of human nature. Here there seems to be a marked contrast between the secular philosophies — the so-called medical-model, psychoanalytical theory, Existentialism and Marxism — and the religious philosophies: Buddhism, Christianity (including the Jewish faith), and Islam. The place of women is inferior to that of men in these religions. It is for theologians to argue whether this follows from the actual doctrines or has simply developed from the institutional structures, but of the facts there can be no doubt. In the West, Christian and Jewish views on women have been affected by the liberal tradition, at least as it applies to health care. But as far as Moslems are concerned there are special problems for those working in obstetrics and gynaecology and some knowledge of what is thought to be respectful would be desirable.

Again, attitudes to suffering and death will vary depending on the view taken of human nature and its place in the scheme of things. On the whole, religious views of suffering will see it as God's will to be borne, and practices such as euthanasia will be strongly discouraged. Other areas likely to be affected by religious views are sexual relationships or abortion practices.

8. CONCLUSION

These views of man and his situation are themselves in very broad terms evaluative − there is no such thing as a value-neutral analysis of the human condition − but they give rise to more specific value-systems. Now, we have said (p. 47) very few people will act consistently or exclusively on one or other of these systems, and there will be values common to all. Nevertheless, each of the views will have its own distinctive flavour and will give rise to characteristic value positions, and reference to those underlying systems may therefore help to explain practical conflicts as to the proper sphere for health care. It is a useful exercise for any health care professional to try to understand the religious or secular beliefs of patients for this is clearly an important part of their well-being.

Chapter 9
ARGUMENTS

1. ASSESSING ARGUMENTS

A knowledge of technical logic is not necessary, and indeed not sufficient, for skill in the use of the arguments which link facts and values. Nevertheless, some awareness of types of argument and what can go wrong with them is helpful to anyone dealing with complex questions of value.

An argument is a related series of statements, one of which is called the conclusion and the others the premises. We argue *from* premises *to* a conclusion, or we support the conclusion with the premises. Logic is the study of the steps from premises to a conclusion, so that to appraise an argument from the logical point of view is to consider whether or not the conclusion does or does not follow from the premises, whether the inference is valid or invalid, or whether the premises entail or imply the conclusion.

Note that logic is not as such concerned with truth or falsity, which are matters of evidence or facts and dealt with by science. Sometimes this point is put by saying that logic is concerned with the *form* of arguments whereas science is concerned with the *content*. Thus a conclusion may still be true even although it does not validly follow from its premises, and equally a conclusion may validly follow from its premises but still be false, if one or both premises are false. For example:

All health care professionals have a mature sense of responsibility.
All nurses have a mature sense of responsibility.
Therefore, all nurses are health care professionals.

The conclusion is true, but the argument is fallacious or invalid in that the premises do not support the conclusion. To bring out what is wrong substitute 'teachers' for 'nurses'. Contrast with the following:

All medical consultants are Conservatives.
All Conservatives support private medicine.
Therefore all medical consultants support private medicine.

The conclusion of this argument is valid, in that it follows from the premises, but it is probably not true because one or both premises are probably false. But if the premises of an argument are true, and the steps valid, then the conclusion must be true.

The first difficulty in logical assessment lies in deciding whether what we are dealing with is intended to be an argument or simply a set of unconnected statements. For example:

The King died and the Queen died.

Are these just two statements simply conjoined with 'and' or is there a hint of a connection? Is the word 'so' implied or not? The *first* thing we must do in appraising arguments then is to be clear whether there is meant to be an argument at all. Usually, but not always, there are words like 'so', 'therefore', 'hence', 'if. . . then. . .', 'either. . . or . . .', 'we can infer that. . .', 'because', 'for the reason that', etc.

The *second* thing we must do is to discover what the conclusion is meant to be. This is not always easy, for sometimes the conclusion comes at the beginning or in the middle of the argument, and sometimes it may not be stated at all but be implied or insinuated. For example:

Some intelligent people do not make good parents, for no selfish people are good parents and some intelligent people are selfish.

In the above example the conclusion comes at the start and is then supported by the clause beginning 'for'. In the next example no conclusion is actually stated but we are clearly meant to draw a conclusion:

A working party consisting of leading churchmen, MPs, and members of the Ethical Committee of the BMA has said that euthanasia is morally wrong.

We are meant to infer 'Therefore euthanasia is wrong'. In an argument it is always important to be clear what one is trying to conclude. Dark hints are not enough!

The *third* thing we must do is to decide whether or not the argument is complete or whether some additional premises are being assumed and should be made explicit. For example:

Nursing is an expertise so it must be based exclusively on science.

This argument is assuming the premise that to be an expertise is to be based exclusively on science. But as soon as the hidden premise is explicitly stated it can be seen to be at least debatable. Are there not expert mountaineers, chess players, and potters, and are their skills based on science?

Some people might retort that mountaineering, etc., *are* sciences, and the discussion of that point would bring out the *fourth* thing we must note in arguing or in assessing arguments — possible ambiguity. Ambiguity is a complex matter, but clearly one source of it is confusion over what we are going to mean by a word. In the above example, there are no doubt senses of 'science' in which we can call mountaineering, playing chess, pottery, or even theology, 'sciences', but these senses are not the same as that in which chemistry, say, is a science. In his *Essays in Pragmatism* William James reports how a dispute arose over ambiguity in the meaning of an expression. A squirrel was clinging to the trunk of a tree, and when someone moved round the tree the squirrel also moved round the trunk so that the trunk was always between itself and the person. There was no dispute that the person went round the tree but did the person also go round the squirrel? Williams James answered as follows:

'Which party is right', I said, 'depends on what you *practically mean* by "going around" the squirrel. If you mean passing from the north of him to the east, then to the south, then to the west, and then to the north of him again, obviously the man does go around him, for he occupies these successive positions.'

'But if on the contrary you mean being first in front of him, then on the right of him, then behind him, then on his left, and finally in front again, it is quite as obvious that the man fails to go round him, for by the compensating movements the squirrel makes, he keeps his belly turned towards the man all the time, and his back turned away. Make the distinction, and there is no occasion for any further dispute.'*

Ambiguity of this kind involves equivocation in the meaning of the words.

Ambiguity can also occur in word order. Some words in particular are liable to confuse if they are not placed carefully in a sentence. For example:

All students are not interested in politics.

This could mean either that no students are interested in politics or that some are not interested. Brevity is another source of ambiguity as in newspaper headlines 'Mother of 13 in Court'. In good argument, then, we must avoid ambiguity or equivocation in the premises or the conclusion.

Ambiguity and equivocation are especially liable to occur in moral arguments, for the reason that the concepts involved are notoriously difficult to define. For example, in his *Utilitarianism* J. S. Mill is committed to defending the view that only happiness in the sense of a sum of pleasure is good as an end in life; everything else is good just as a means to happiness in this sense. To the objection that surely health, virtue, knowledge of science, appreciation of the arts, etc., are also good as ends, Mill replies that they are indeed good as ends because they are 'part of happiness'. But happiness now means something different from what it did at the start. No doubt we can use happiness both in a narrow sense as a sum of pleasures and also in a wide sense as whatever it is we regard as desirable as an end in life, but we cannot use it in both senses at once in the same argument.†

---

*James, William. (1948). *Essays in Pragmatism*, p. 141. Hafner, New York.
†Mill, J. S. *Utilitarianism*, Chapter 4.

We come now, *fifth*, to the distinction between two kinds of argument, called deductive and inductive arguments. Deductive arguments proceed from general or universal premises to a particular or singular conclusion, or to a general conclusion. For example:

> All social workers vote Labour.
> Fred is a social worker.
> Therefore Fred will vote Labour.

or

> No Labour voters believe in private medicine.
> All social workers vote Labour.
> Therefore no social workers believe in private medicine.

Inductive arguments proceed from the particular or singular to the general or universal, or deal with frequencies or probabilities. For example:

> Several groups of typical social workers vote Labour.
> Therefore, all social workers vote Labour.

or

> Fred has a clean driving licence, a full no-claims bonus, and a police driver's certificate.
> Therefore, you'll be safe if you're driven by Fred.

We can say that deductive arguments are such that (a) if the premises are true the conclusion must be true, and (b) the conclusion contains no new information that was not already implicit in the premises. Inductive arguments are such that (a) if the premises are true the conclusion is probably but not necessarily true, and (b) the conclusion contains information not present even implicitly in the premises. Inductive arguments are common in the sciences where the accumulation of evidence makes conclusions increasingly probable. In moral debate, however, deductive forms of argument are much more common and we shall concentrate on these.

Sixth, it is important to be clear on what logicians call the 'logical status' of the conclusion, or the premises, otherwise we cannot be sure that appropriate methods of argument have been used. Some statements are what logicians call analytic, conceptual or necessary. Definitions are of this sort. For example, 'Bachelors are unmarried men'. Some statements are empirical, factual, or contingent. For example, 'Most consultants play golf'. Some statements are normative or evaluative. Moral judgements are of this kind. For example, 'Patients ought to see their records'. It is important that the premises supporting the conclusion be of the appropriate kind. For example:

> Doctors ought not to condone euthanasia (or abortion) since the medical profession exists by definition to heal.

The conclusion of this argument (that doctors ought not to condone euthanasia or abortion) is clearly a moral judgement. But moral judgements cannot be *established* by definitions; it is always logically possible to judge that doctors ought to act differently. Consider a second example:

> Inducing labour in childbirth is a good policy since it is widely practised.

This is an attempt to settle what is a good policy (an evaluative matter) by appealing to what is in fact done. But it is not logically possible to settle what ought to be done by appealing to what is in fact done, although clearly some knowledge of what in fact is done would always be relevant to settling what is a good policy.

2. THE STRUCTURE OF MORAL ARGUMENT

Moral arguments often have an underlying form. They have a *major premise*, which is some moral rule or principle, a *minor premise*, which is a statement of fact connecting the situation under discussion with the rule, and a *conclusion* which tells us what we ought or ought not to do, or what would be morally right or wrong. For example:

Major	It is wrong (one ought not) to deceive someone
premise	about a matter which is important for his future
	welfare.

Minor	Failure to disclose to Jones the full facts about his
premise	disease deceives him about a matter which is
	important for his future welfare.

Conclusion	Therefore, it is wrong to fail to disclose to Jones
	the full facts about his disease.

Debate about such arguments can be directed at either the minor premise (i.e. the alleged facts) or at the major premise (the rule). As far as the minor premise is concerned it might be maintained that the alleged facts are inaccurate, mistaken, incomplete, or not fully known, or that they do not really constitute a case to which the rule applies. In our example it might be maintained that Jones *was* told, or that he was too ill to take in what was said, or that it was not yet certain that he had the disease, or that a failure to go into the full facts (which he would *not* understand) does not really constitute a case of deception.

It is obvious that debates over the minor premise will often involve questions of scientific knowledge and uncertainty of the sort we have already discussed (Chapter 2), but less obvious that discussions of the facts will often involve moral judgements. It is a matter of moral judgement whether or not the absence of a full disclosure of the facts constitutes a case of 'deception' if the patient has been informed to the extent that is common practice among the professional peer groups. For example, let us suppose that there is a 1 per cent chance of a serious side-effect of some procedure. Has the patient been 'deceived' if this fact is not communicated? The answer to this question is not one of *fact*, but of moral opinion.

Again, dispute over the minor premise might be *conceptual*. For example, suppose the patient presents with a skin problem which in a technical scientific sense is 'cancer', but is of a kind which is easily and successfully treatable. Is this a case of cancer in the patient's or layman's perception of that concept? Would it not in fact deceive him *more* to tell him that he had cancer (although this is technically true)? Clearly, then, in disputes over the minor premise, the main discussion may be over the facts, but moral and conceptual judgements may also be interwoven.

Turning now to the major premise we find that disputes over it might again be moral, factual, or conceptual, although the emphasis here will be on morality. For example, it might be maintained that whereas it is wrong to deceive people about matters affecting their own future welfare it is also wrong to give them information which will upset them at a crucial stage in an illness. At this point in the discussion other moral principles might be invoked. For example, it might be said that what is really wrong about deception is not that it is detrimental to welfare (which, as a matter of fact, it sometimes is and sometimes is not) but that it is an offence against autonomy, and that respect for the autonomy of a person is morally more important than concern for his welfare. In other words, in disputes about the major premise in a moral argument we connect our judgements with higher-order principles.

To sum up this account of moral judgement we can say that moral disputes typically break out over particular cases – whether we ought or ought not to treat a given patient in a given way. Facts, concepts, and rules are always involved with different degrees of importance in different disputes. Typically we might argue that X is wrong for reasons A, B, C and assume that all cases of A, B, C are wrong. Someone might disagree on the grounds that (a) reasons A, B, C do not here apply (we are wrong in our facts or concepts); or (b) not all cases of A, B, C are wrong (other rules apply). In the end, however, we shall find that all the rules of the morality of health care can be seen as applications of the broad principles we stated in Chapter 4, and ultimately instances of respect for the autonomous individual.

We have outlined the typical framework of moral argument, but within that framework moves can be made which are illogical, although not always easy to avoid unless we are aware of them. Let us now turn to some of these.

3. COMMON TYPES OF ARGUMENT, MAINLY BAD

1.   The first kind of bad argument we shall mention is called 'begging the question'. This consists in assuming in the argument the truth of what we are meant to be proving. It is especially liable to be found in moral reasoning where the protagonists in the argument are so convinced of the correctness of their position that they assume it in all their arguments. For example, in abortion debates it is begging the question to say that what is wrong with abortion is that it involves murder, if we are meant to assume that only persons can be murdered and what is at stake is the question of whether or not the fetus is reasonably to be called a person. A slightly different form of question-begging occurs in the following exchange:

A: No serious musician likes jazz.
B: But Menuhin likes jazz.
A: He can't be a serious musician then.

The point here is that objections to a view are being disallowed by the device of interpreting them in terms of the concepts of the thesis that is in dispute.

Another form of question-begging uses the 'All right-thinking Americans' approach.

All right-thinking Americans know that national sovereignty must be protected against the inroads of international organizations like the UN.

Any American who disagrees is immediately disqualified because he cannot be right-thinking. This begs the question. Similarly, beware of the argument which suggests that 'All *true* Christians believe. . .' or 'All experienced nurses know. . .'

2.   A second fallacious kind of argument involves a confusion between questions of the origins of something, which are matters of psychology, sociology, history, or some other natural or social science, and questions of the justification of something, which require argument and rational assessment. For example,

it may be urged against a person's moral judgement, that he is making it only because he is influenced by someone else, only because he belongs to a certain social class, only because of a bad experience he had, etc. Women suffer in this way. It is often hinted or asserted that they believe what they do just because it is 'the time of the month', because they need a boyfriend, etc. The point is that all these allegations might well be true, but they are irrelevant to the question of whether what is asserted is justifiable or not. Suppose it is true, to take another example, that our moral consciences are just the voices of our parents: this in no way affects the validity or otherwise of our moral judgement on a given issue. Sometimes this is called the 'genetic fallacy'.

3. A connected sort of bad argument, or non-argument, is the *ad hominem* kind. Those against abortion are often referred to as 'emotional', as if that disposed of their views, whereas those in favour of it might be referred to as a 'pressure group' or in some other way which suggests that they do not really have a rational argument for their case. There are numerous terms of rhetoric for and against issues. For example, views or their supporters can be denigrated with terms like 'trendy', 'ivory-tower', 'long-haired', 'unrealistic', 'immature', 'natural', or 'unnatural'. What these terms have in common is that they are all quite irrelevant to the rational criticism of any point of view.

4. Appeals to authority are of doubtful worth in moral debate. This is an age of experts, and expert witnesses are often appealed to about moral questions. But there is no reason why a consultant or an MP or a professor or a bishop or a round-the-world-yachtsman should have a better view on moral questions than the rest of us. Prominent people may be experts in their own line of business, but moral questions do not require expertise of that sort. It is true that the views of someone with a rich and varied experience of life may be more worth having than someone who has lived a life of narrow confinement. But often distinguished people have achieved their distinction at the cost of a life dedicated to the pursuit of narrow goals. Judges, for example, who often pronounce on moral questions, are not noted for their

sympathy for women, or in general for the width of their experience. Be that as it may, moral questions cannot be settled by appeal to authority, and this is especially relevant to health care problems where, as we have argued throughout, matters of moral and scientific substance are hard to distinguish.

5. It is easy to be misled in an argument by technical-sounding words, which may not say anything at all. Molière makes fun of this when a character is said to go to sleep because of 'dormitive power'.
Another example is the following:

> Frogs can survive either on land or in water. This is due to the fact that they are characteristically amphibious.

Clearly, the word 'amphibious' simply repeats the stated facts and does not explain them.

6. Doubtful analogies are a source of weak argumentation. Sometimes, of course, there is a real and appreciated problem about how far it is scientifically legitimate to extrapolate from one population or system to another. For example:

> Experiments confirm that when rats are overcrowded they become aggressive. This indicates that overcrowding in our cities may be one of the major causes of violence in industrial society.

The whole scientific issue of drug testing on animals raises similar issues. Those are really problems of extrapolation. But sometimes there are more serious problems of argument with analogies properly so-called. For example:

> War can never be a means of bringing about peace. If you plant wheat, you get wheat. If you plant thistles, you won't get strawberries. Likewise, if you plant hatred and killing you can't expect peace and justice. Fighting for peace is just like fornicating for chastity.

The use of striking analogies of this sort is the stock-in-trade of evangelical moralists. They can illuminate a problem, but by concentrating our attention on one aspect of it they can also mislead.

7. It is important to be aware that what is true of individuals is not necessarily true of the collective or group as a whole. For example:

> Man is a fighting animal; therefore the nation, being a community of men, must be a fighting unit (Churchill).

Equally, what is true of a group as a whole is not necessarily true of every member. The National Health Service may be open to criticism, but it does not follow that every member of it is open to criticism.

8. In moral debates it is not uncommon to find the 'slippery slope' argument. In this kind of argument it is agreed that doing A may not, perhaps, be wrong. But it is asserted that doing A will lead to doing B and C, and that we shall reach a point at which we all accept the doing of X which is wrong. Therefore we ought not to do A. For example, in the debate on experimentation on the human embryo some people have argued that, while it may not in itself be wrong to experiment on the human embryo provided that the experiments are not carried out after 14 days, to condone such experimentation will weaken deep inhibitions and set us off down a slope leading to experiments on the embryo at 28 days, the brain-damaged at any age, the senile. . . In assessing this kind of argument we must be sure that there is a slope, and that the slide is not stoppable before we reach what is wrong. Otherwise, it does not seem a strong argument against doing what is admitted to be morally good.

There is another form of the 'slippery slope' argument which can be stronger. This is the argument that if you once move out of some accepted position there seems no non-arbitrary way of stopping the move to other positions. For example, suppose a couple wish to have a small wedding. They might achieve this by asking as guests only members of their own immediate families. If they once ask a few non-family friends there is no non-arbitrary way of excluding a large number of other friends.

This kind of problem can occur in the just allocation of scarce resources.

9. It is controversial to say that the 'double effect' argument is a bad one, for many people regard it as effective. It is used particularly in some religious contexts. The argument stresses the moral importance of intentions, and draws a sharp distinction between intended *ends* of action and foreseen but unintended *consequences*. For example, if I am attacked I am morally permitted to use force to defend myself; 'defending myself' is the intended and morally permitted end of my actions. In defending myself I may correctly foresee the unintended consequence that my assailant will be injured or killed. But I am not morally guilty of his injury or death (provided the force used was not excessive) because that was not my intention.

The argument can be used in various health care contexts. For example, let us assume that euthanasia is morally wrong. The double effect argument can be used to justify a massive dosage of pain-killing drugs for someone dying of cancer who is in great pain. The morally permitted intention is to relieve pain, and it is a foreseen but unintended consequence that the patient dies. Again, even if we assume that abortion is always wrong, we might still operate on the uterus of a pregnant women to remove a malignant growth. The death of the fetus would be foreseen, but not intended.

In assessing the double effect argument note first that it assumes that there are certain sorts of policy which are always wrong in themselves, such as abortion, suicide or euthanasia. Without this assumption there is no *need* for double effect arguments. But not everyone would agree that certain sorts of action are always wrong, or right, *whatever the consequences*.

Second, the argument assumes that we can always distinguish between what is intended and what is merely foreseen, and that such a distinction is always morally relevant. But, if an obstetrician operates on the uterus of a pregnant but seriously ill woman, can we distinguish between saying on the one hand that the intention was to save the life of the woman and a foreseen but unintended consequence was the death of the fetus, and on the other hand that the intention was to procure an abortion in order to save the life of the woman? And supposing we could draw this distinction, is it morally relevant in any case? If Captain Oates walked into the snow it does not seem to matter morally whether we say he intended to walk on his own to prevent himself from being a burden to his companions and foresaw his certain death, or whether we say that he intended to commit suicide to save his companions. Either way it was a gallant action. Only those who wish to maintain that suicide is always wrong whatever the consequences will prefer the first description.

The double effect argument is useful only to those holding absolutist principles and the danger of the argument is that it encourages moral dishonesty.

Logic is a practical subject, just as morality is practical. We therefore include some examples of moral argument for discussion.

4. EXERCISES

1. Common types of moral argument

The following are often used in moral arguments. Think of medical or other contexts in which you have used them or have heard them used. How far do you consider them to be convincing in their various contexts?

1. 'Think of what would happen if everyone did it.'
2. 'Well, you wouldn't like it, would you?'
3. 'My conscience wouldn't allow it.'
4. 'It hurts; that's why it's wrong.'
5. 'It won't do any good to tell her, so why bother?'
6. 'It must be all right, everyone does it.'
7. 'When in Rome, do as the Romans do!'
8. 'I always put "number one" first. You're a fool if you don't.'
9. 'Those who know about these things say it's all right.'
10. 'People weren't meant to do that sort of thing.'

11. 'It's against human nature.'
12. 'It's only human nature.'
13. 'It's against the law.'
14. 'You are taking it too seriously − it was just a joke.'
15. 'I only took a few.'
16. 'Nobody is much interested whether you do it or not.'
17. 'He doesn't know any better.'
18. 'It is for his own good.'
19. 'It's just your tough luck.'
20. 'It's for the good of others.'

2. Lies

Identify and evaluate the arguments in the following passages for and against not telling lies. Do not write a general discourse about lies, but pick out (as a, b, c, etc.) the specific arguments and comment on them briefly. Be alert to the possibility that some of the arguments a speaker uses may be inconsistent with others he/she uses.

Frank: Telling lies is wrong in itself. It's an abuse of the gift of speech − telling lies can hardly be the purpose of speech, can it? It's one of those things that people in all times and places have held to be wrong, and it's easy to see why they've condemned it: if everyone went around telling lies, society would break down. Obviously, then, you mustn't lie. Lies poison relations between people, and every lie pushes us further down the slippery slope to total distrust and isolation. It's all very well to say, 'Tell a lie if the consequences justify doing so', but you can never know the consequences your acts will have. *You* wouldn't like to be lied to, would you? Well, then, don't tell lies yourself. We *need* to know the truth − how otherwise can we live our lives as free and responsible people? To be lied to is really to have your freedom denied and your human dignity affronted − we h..ve a right to be told the truth.

Anne: Telling the truth may often be right and desirable, but people can make a silly fetish of it. Someone whose conscience would never let him tell a lie is in the grip of a silly obsession like people who can't bring themselves to step on the cracks in the pavement — they need to see reason. Lies are often harmless — what harm does it do to tell someone you liked their performance in a play, even if you thought they were awful? — and often beneficial, even necessary; a doctor may know it would utterly crush someone to know the truth, and if we tell a thug where his intended victim is, we're indirectly responsible for the victim's smashed-in face. If other people are profiting by lying, getting welfare benefits, say, by giving false information, you're simply denying yourself your share if you don't lie too, and that's silly. Anyway, truth isn't always attainable and may not even exist. People see the world in different ways, truth can be a subjective thing, it can be sheer tyranny to insist that your vision is the truth and another's is false.

3. Responsibility and excuses

We have argued that a person is responsible for his actions if he has the freedom and the knowledge to do them. It follows from this that a person is morally excused if it can be shown that on given occasions he either could not help doing as he did because he was in some way compelled, or in some way he did not know what he was doing. For example, if someone is pushed and as a result breaks a valuable vase then, whatever the legal liability, we do not feel that he was morally to blame, because 'he couldn't help it'. There are, however, more complicated cases in which the compulsion is alleged to be psychological, an 'irresistible impulse'. For example, it is sometimes said that premenstrual tension or menopausal conditions can compel actions and therefore count as excuses. How far do you agree?

Again, there is a sort of compulsion called 'duress'. The clearest case of this is that in which the gunman threatens death unless the jewels are handed over. This is not quite like other cases of compulsion in that there is still, in a sense, a choice — sometimes choosing death may be the right course — but the action cannot really be called voluntary, for no one would have chosen it were it not for the duress. For example, fear or suffering may render someone incapable of choice. Is this duress or another sort of compulsion? How far do pain and suffering render patients incapable of consenting to treatment?

Lack of knowledge excuses in clear cases, as when a person could not possibly have known what he was doing. But there is a range of difficult cases in which it is arguable that a person's lack of knowledge amounts to some sort of moral negligence. Perhaps the nurse should have known that moving the patient or not moving the patient would be a cause of pain or discomfort.

The usual excuse, based on a plea of lack of knowledge or ignorance or mistake, refers to a matter of fact — that the solution in the syringe was the wrong one, perhaps, that the accused claims he could not possibly have known. But can there be moral ignorance? For example, a doctor in his private life may be aware that telling lies, rudeness, lack of punctuality, etc., are wrong, but be unaware that what he does in his professional life comes under that description. Is this lack of awareness morally culpable or not?

PART 2

Chapter 10
LEARNING AND TEACHING MORAL VALUES

1. MORAL AND OTHER SORTS OF KNOWLEDGE

The question whether virtue can be taught is an old one which was much discussed by Plato.* We have tried to show in Chapter 2 that some of the complexities of the question are due to the fact that moral knowledge is not one kind of knowledge but is a compound. In explaining this, as we saw in Chapter 1, philosophers sometimes distinguish between factual knowledge, practical knowledge, and knowledge of values and attitudes. Factual knowledge is clearly important for moral knowledge and decision-making. This is particularly true in the field of health care. It is impossible for a doctor or a nurse to make a humane and wise decision about how to treat or care for a patient in the absence of a sound basis of knowledge deriving from the natural and the social sciences; and it is equally impossible to implement that decision without the practical skills. To the extent that moral knowledge involves information and skills, it is clearly learnable and teachable, and the vast proportion of health care studies are concerned with just those.

But we also saw in Chapter 2 that moral knowledge and decision-making are not completely reducible to knowledge of facts, even facts about human behaviour, and morally good conduct is not just a matter of skills or techniques. It is a question

Republic; Meno; Protagoras.

of interest and importance whether, and if so how, the remaining element — morality pure and simple — can be learned and taught. Before embarking on the question we must also remind ourselves of another aspect of the matter. Values do not follow from facts in any straightforward way. How then do we connect the facts of the natural and social sciences with moral values or 'oughts'? As we have seen, the answer is by using various sorts of argument. Learning and teaching morality therefore require some ability to follow and appraise arguments. This is not, of course, to say that the saint must be a logician! It is to say, however, that a certain competence in dealing with arguments is a help in separating the relevant from the irrelevant, or the genuinely convincing from the merely rhetorical. Teaching and learning about morality therefore involve facts, skills, values, and arguments. In this chapter, let us look at ways of teaching and learning about values or morality.

2. LEARNING AND TEACHING MORALITY

We are none of us beginners in this. From infancy people learn and are taught morality by parents, schoolteachers, friends, colleagues, or television programmes. In that sense, then, learning about morality as a medical or nursing student is not like learning about biochemistry, where no previous knowledge can be presupposed. Moreover, our values change as we grow older; they are not fixed. But how can values be taught?

As a start in answering this question it is instructive to consider the traditional way of doing it and to consider its defects. The traditional method — although 'method' is perhaps the wrong term since it was never fully explicit — involved two stages. In the first stage, which usually took place early in the student's college or university years, some important and senior person would arrive and give a lecture or two on the relevant 'Code of Ethics' and then disappear and never be seen again. This had the effect of suggesting that ethics was something exalted and unconnected with one's everyday moral concerns.

The second stage took place during clinical teaching and the idea was that the student acquired an 'ethical' grasp from observing the practice of an experienced professional. Just as the novice surgeon or the nursing student picks up knowledge and techniques from watching an experienced practitioner so ethics was expected to be absorbed. This stage, of course, presupposes that the senior's practice is exemplary, which it may not be, and that there is no room for other ways of looking at moral questions.

The basic assumption, common to both stages of the traditional method, is that explicit or implicit instruction must always be given exclusively by a senior member of the relevant profession − thus reinforcing the idea that 'ethics' is an occult matter the mysteries of which are not for the layman or the inexperienced student. Criticism by outsiders of current practices is seen as 'doctor bashing' or 'nurse bashing', and the idea that the professional could sometimes learn from outsiders, or from juniors in the profession, is not thinkable.

This description is no doubt exaggerated but has sufficient truth in it to warrant some suggestions for other ways of proceeding. We should like to suggest that the following factors are important for improving the teaching of morality in health care contexts, and therefore for improving health care. Attention must be given to:

(1) the integration of the teaching environment;
(2) the content of what is taught;
(3) how it is taught;
(4) who teaches it;
(5) the example set in the hospital or any other care environment.

1.   Whereas it is important that there should be lectures or other formal ways of teaching ethics in college or university this teaching will come to nothing unless it is explicitly integrated with the practice experiences of the student and is seen to be relevant. The teachers at each stage must know and refer to what has already been said, and above all the practitioners must

take up relevant points and illustrate them. There should be co-ordination.

2,3. The content and method of teaching will depend on resources but it is important to encourage *critical* discussion of a *realistic* sort. Thus, students might be asked to discuss cases and then to say what they would have done. Whereas much of the material for such discussions will involve case-histories and moral philosophy, it is important to remember that novels, poems, plays, or films can make a large impact on a student and develop the intuitive understanding we have stressed throughout the book. Heaven forbid that literature should be studied only because it is useful, but a study of literature is *educative* because it is able to provide insight into the particularity of situations. Whereas science, including social science, proceeds by induction from specific instances to generalized (often idealized) patterns, literature explores unique situations which may include conflicts of value of the kind discussed elsewhere in this book. It thereby enables us to acquire insights into universal human predicaments. Study of this sort is as relevant to the career of a doctor, nurse, or social worker as is the study of highly abstract systematic sociology.

4. Turning from literature to the fourth of the factors we have noted as important in moral education – the matter of *who* should be involved – we have found that it is helpful if the enterprise is a co-operative one with people outside the particular profession. For the professionals to do it all themselves gives a recipe for conservatism and whitewash, but if the classes are taken entirely by others then the students may not regard them with sufficient seriousness. Co-operation is essential, although not always easy to arrange. Moral philosophers, social scientists and lawyers have an important place in teaching; so do patients and relatives who can contribute a quite different slant on moral problems.

5. The fifth factor in moral education is the influence of seniors. Students will learn just as much or more from what is actually done in the real situation as from what is said. The

teamwork between professionals of more than one discipline, stressed in later chapters, can be effective as an example in learning and teaching moral values.

Let us now consider in more detail two methods of introducing discussion of moral issues in health care. They are not, of course, exhaustive or exclusive, and indeed the employment of a combination of them would be desirable.

3. THE USE OF CASE-HISTORIES, QUESTIONS, OR STATEMENTS

This is the most common method and it appeals to students because actual cases can be used and this creates the atmosphere of realism which is essential if medical, nursing, or other health care students are to treat the subject seriously. Certainly it is important that cases should be related to general principles and broad lessons drawn from such discussion, but without the clinical details students will lose interest. There are, however, three common problems raised by students in the discussions provoked by case-histories or practical examples. The first is the 'it depends' response. This view is that there are so many variables which are not given, and which would be required to make a decision, that it is not worth trying. The response would 'depend' on so many things that it is not possible even to discuss the issue.

The second problem is that the responses are so individual that decision is irrelevant. This view makes the point that the subjective nature of the responses means that particular views on a topic are unlikely to change in a brief discussion.

The third problem is that before the questions or case-histories are discussed more professional knowledge or experience is required. The argument here is that only when you become a consultant, ward sister, etc., will you have sufficient background to tackle such questions. What, then, is the point in trying?

These problems are important, and need to be considered further. Suppose you are asked to discuss the statement 'Patients over the age of 70 should not be resuscitated'. Clearly, whether you agree or disagree with the statement *will* depend on many factors. The point of the exercise is to get you to think of the circumstances under which you would agree, or not. For example, you might agree to a resuscitation policy under the following conditions:

'Patients who have previously been well, and with no other illnesses, with a good social environment and a supportive family'

and you could list conditions under which you would disagree with a resuscitation policy, such as:

'Multiple medical problems, no family support, etc.'

Equally, however, you could disagree with the approach that there *should* be guide-lines for resuscitation, and maintain that it is morally wrong to have guide-lines on this. You might broaden the discussion to raise the question as to who should make the decision.

In other words, the reason for giving you such statements is to make you question the assumption behind them, and to help to clarify your own thoughts and attitudes behind your response. We have discussed some of the complexities of resuscitation in Chapter 5, and more generally it is important to be familiar with the structure and pitfalls of moral argument, (see Chapter 9).

The second concern about such statements is that responses are always personalized, and that within groups there could always be differences of opinion. But the reason for discussion is not necessarily to achieve a consensus; it can also be to allow individual views to be heard, and to make participants aware that there may be more than one view on the subject. This is in order that:

1. You can be clearer about your own views.
2. You can understand the views of others, whether they be patients, relatives, or staff.
3. You can consider your response to those with whom you disagree.

Point 3 is important. In your professional life you *will* disagree with others. How are you to deal with this? Group discussions give an opportunity for testing your reactions to disagreement.

The third concern often voiced in discussion is that it is impossible to answer many of the questions raised because you do not have sufficient clinical experience. This view makes the assumption that greater experience, status, and knowledge can help to answer such questions. It also assumes that at a certain stage in one's career, the answers to ethical and moral questions become obvious. Now while there is no doubt that increasing clinical experience can change particular views, one only has to consider the differences in views among senior members of professional groups to realize that experience alone will not ensure a consensus of opinion. Finally, you should remember that you may be faced with many of the situations described *before* you reach some elevated status and you will require to have a view now on these matters.

New knowledge, new techniques, and new information are continually becoming available and therefore professional experience will change with time. Most clinical decisions are based on information which is less than complete. Assumptions are made, and decisions made on the basis of probabilities. There may be no certainty as to the outcome of a particular course of action. To delay making moral decisions until all possible factual information is available is to misunderstand the nature of clinical decision-making.

The conclusion then is that statements and case-histories should be seen as 'triggers' to discussion, and as stimuli for thought. They are essentially 'coat-pegs' on which to hang concepts and views.

4. USING LITERATURE AND THE ARTS

The initial impetus to the health care ethics movement came from a fusion of medical concerns with moral philosophy, and that is still the main source of energy. When moral philosophy dominates, however, the discussion can easily become too abstract. One antidote to abstraction is to use literature and the arts.

What can medicine learn from the arts? It is a matter for the theorists to discuss whether the arts ought to set out to be didactic, but it is in fact the case that good art inevitably gives rise to moral questions. It is not that the arts present us with some unrealistic idea, but rather that they explore the many facets of our ambiguous views on illness. When this happens, we find ourselves reconsidering the quality of our care.

If the arts generate moral questions they also develop our capacities to answer them. Once again it is tempting to follow the philosophers and think of the resolution of moral questions in terms of the application of principles supported by rational argument. As we have stressed, principles and logic certainly have their place, but the arts can extend our imaginations and deepen our sympathies and these capacities are also essential to the wise and humane doctor and the caring nurse. The point here is that philosophers, like biological and social scientists, must stand back from the phenomena and present their accounts in detached prose style. On the other hand, the arts involve us directly and make us vividly and emotionally aware of what it is like to be in the situation which the philosopher and social scientist discuss, of what it means to be ill oneself, or to be a relative or helper of someone who is ill. In this way the arts develop sympathy of the passive or empathetic kind. Now, passive sympathy easily generates motivation to act, and active sympathy, however well-meaning, can be blind, clumsy, or humiliating unless it is informed by a sensitive understanding of particular situations or relationships. But the arts have this other aspect, too: namely, that they can inform sympathy or give it a cognitive shaping. In other words, the arts can develop our perceptions of the complex nature of needs, and inspire an appropriate compassion.

Caring for those in need can, of course, raise questions of the meaning of life, of the tragedy and tears, and sometimes the comic absurdity, built into human relationships. Such questions inevitably arise in medical situations and require some sort of answer if the life of professional care is to seem worthwhile. The arts can approach these questions with an immediacy lacking in the abstractions of philosophy or social sciences. Moreover, this immediacy can provide a catharsis, a relief from pent-up emotion and tensions, through tears and laughter.

The arts also develop our self-perceptions. The treatment of doctors and nurses by non-medical writers can here be of interest, often salutary interest, to the professions. Doctors are so used to being in positions of power over patients that it is good for them to be made aware that they are also figures of fun. This can encourage a realistic sense of proportion, and many doctors appreciate this. But whereas Chaucer's Doctour of Physik is a portrait tinged with irony, George Eliot's Lydgate is presented as an ideal with which many doctors can still identify – concerned with patients but also pursuing scientific research. He represents the self they still feel to be their true self, despite the cynicism engendered by a life of committee meetings.

Communication is of central importance in health care. This is one to which the arts can make a major contribution. For example, literature focuses attention on language, on the connotations and resonances of words used to describe or express feelings and fears. Painting, on the other hand, brings out the non-verbal ways in which feelings or attitudes can be expressed. Take, for example, the sympathetic portrayal of the doctor in the painting 'The Doctor' by Sir Luke Fildes, which hangs in the Tate Gallery in London. As an illustration of the doctor–patient relationship this has an eloquent sensitivity which communicates itself more directly than a treatise. No amount of science, social science, or philosophy can succeed in conveying with the subtlety and infinite variety of the arts this basic aspect of human relationships and therefore of doctor–patient relationships.

So far we have been maintaining that the enjoyment of the arts can at the same time enrich the practice of health care by generating moral questions, by stretching the imagination and deepening the sympathies, by providing a catharsis for the tensions and emotions produced in health care practice, by increasing self-awareness and restoring lost ideals, and by focusing attention on communication. This recapitulation enables us to make explicit the central theme which unifies the arts approach to health care – it is that health care is itself an art. Despite the enormous developments in the sciences relevant to health care – and these are just about all the sciences and social sciences – the simple truth remains: doctors and nurses treat patients and not disease-entities. No matter how well-informed in the sciences doctors and nurses are nowadays obliged to become, the actual treatment of patients has the characteristics of art, and can be sensitive or insensitive as art can be. This thesis, once upon a time widely recognized in health care education, is now sufficiently contentious to require some further explanation and defence.

First, as we argued in Chapter 2, science by its very essence is concerned with the general, the repeatable elements in nature including human nature; but health care, using science, is concerned with the particularity, the uniqueness of individual patients. In its concern with the particular and the unique health care resembles the arts.

Second, in its concentration on the repeatable patterns and laws of nature science must of necessity be impersonal; it records the meaningless processes which would continue whether we were there or not to participate. Medicine on the other hand must be concerned with what illness and disease mean for a given patient. This is not to say that disease has a meaning – diseases are impersonal like any other processes which can be understood by science – but it is to say that diseases have meanings for patients. One and the same disease might have quite a different meaning for two patients and therefore different treatments might be appropriate. The arts are the vehicles through which human beings articulate the meanings of their lives.

Third, health care and the arts are each concerned with healing, with bringing about wholeness. This is the most important point: the artist attends nature as the doctor or nurse attend the patient. Each must be attentive in looking and listening and encouraging a response.

There will, of course, be objections to what has been claimed for health care and the arts. We have claimed that the practice of health care is an art, although an art informed by science. It may be objected that at best it has been established only that health care has some features in common with the arts; perhaps it is better viewed as a craft than an art. This objection will not be discussed, for it is sufficient for our purposes if the resemblances between the practice of medicine and the arts are noted. They certainly exist in striking parallels if not identities.

A second objection is that the insight and understanding achieved through the arts is, of all disreputable things, un-scientific (and therefore in some sense superficial or spurious). Someone pressing this objection would see the point of the arts as simply giving pleasure 'to them as likes that kind of thing'. Now the arts certainly give pleasure, but enjoyment can have a deep structure; pushpin is not as good as poetry, at least if one wants more than the pleasure of a momentary diversion. Is it true, then, that the insight or understanding achieved through the arts is unscientific?

It is certainly non-scientific, because, as we have maintained, scientific understanding is concerned with patterns, with what is repeatable, whereas the kind of understanding which comes from the arts does not arise from what is repeatable but is unique to each situation. But it does not follow from the point that this sort of understanding is non-scientific either that it cannot be based on any evidence or that there is no way of testing it. The evidence will be patients' own accounts of how they see their situations or problems, and testing one's understanding of their situations is a matter of, for example, gauging their reactions to further questions. A knowledge of social science might be a help here, but it is just as likely to be an impediment, because it will encourage the doctor or nurse to see unique individuals and their problems in terms of general categories and labels.

The term 'folk psychology' is sometimes invoked to disparage the kind of insights and understanding which come from the arts. The assumption seems to be that imaginative writers and artists are attempting to do crudely and unsystematically what modern psychologists do in a sophisticated and rigorous manner. This assumption needs only to be stated for its absurdity to be seen. Imaginative writers or artists are not attempting to write systematic treatises on human behaviour, although this does not mean that what they write is not, in another sense, psychology. It is the term 'folk' that is objectionable in the expression, with its suggestions of unlearned naïvety. But the arts abound in refined, accurate, and sensitive analyses of human beings and their relationships and need not be at all simple-minded.

It is important to insist that we can indeed learn from the arts, while denying that it teaches us by generalizing from experience. The important question is not 'Can we learn from the arts?' but 'How do we learn from the arts?' The answer to the question thus re-formulated is that we learn by imaginative identification with the situations or characters depicted, and by having our imaginations stretched through being made to enter into unfamiliar situations or to see points of view other than our own. Learning of this kind is generative of a deep understanding which is essential to humane nursing and doctoring; it is the key to achieving the 'whole person understanding' which some critics find missing in the practice of health care.

5. USING PART 2

An important thesis of this book is that morality can be taught and learned, and that values, opinions, and attitudes can change. They will not change, however, if individuals or teams do not actively engage in discussing such matters. There is good evidence that, granted discussion and reflection, such things do change with time. To take a non-medical example, think of your own taste in music or clothes and ask yourself how this has altered over the years. As we grow older, our values change. This book, however, is not just about change. Even if your own moral values do not change after reading this book we hope that you will be clearer in your own mind as to *why* the particular values you hold are important to you and, further, that if required you could defend these values with cogent and logical arguments.

Part 2 of this book deals with a series of practical issues which illustrate more concretely the problems in morality faced by health care professionals. It will be remembered that in the

Introduction we distinguished three senses of ethics, as moral philosophy, as practical morality, and as professional codes. In Part 1 we were dealing with health care issues from the perspective of moral philosophy, and now in Part 2 we are going to approach them from the other end — from the practical perspective of those who must make the decision in wards or surgeries. Having given some structure to moral thinking in Part 1 we hope to look at some of the details in Part 2; and at the end of Part 2 to have a briefer discussion of professional codes.

Since opinion is likely to be divided on many of the issues raised, it will not be possible to provide an instant solution to moral problems. That would be to deny the whole concept of this book. Rather, we shall discuss various issues and present to the reader case-histories or clinical situations, together with a series of questions which the reader must answer for him or herself.

The book may be used by individual students, by groups or classes, or by teachers. Whoever uses the book, it is essential that there is involvement and that active discussion takes place. We learn from each other as much as from books.

For individual students: As you read through the next few chapters pay special attention to the case-histories, questions, and comments. Keep a notebook handy and where possible actually commit yourself to paper. Think, if you can, of more than one answer to the questions, or of other questions to answer. Make sure that the views you hold can be sustained by argument. Refer back to Part 1 of the book to clarify points and obtain additional information.

For groups or classes: It is hoped that the numerous examples given in this section of the book will provide the basis for group discussions. It is important that all students are involved in this, and where possible that the teaching should be on a multi-professional basis. In this way the special expertise, knowledge, and values of different groups can be used.

For teachers: The examples given in this book can be taken and altered to suit particular local needs, or professional interests.

They can be prepared as overhead displays or as written hand-outs. It is essential to encourage participation by the student; even within a large class discussion is possible, especially if students are divided quickly into groups of about four to six, given a problem to discuss among themselves for about five minutes, and then asked what conclusions they have reached. Many of the examples could also be used for project work by the class.

For all readers: The key is to review the information, the evidence and the opinion, before logically analysing the situation and making a decision. In a short book it is impossible to give all the arguments for and against a particular problem. For this reason an additional task of the reader is to amass more information or evidence. Clearly, this must be a continual process as public, professional, and personal attitudes and values change. For this reason it is important that the personal answers given are reviewed at intervals in the light of experience. It is important to recall that one of the objectives of this book is to allow the reader to determine his or her own approach to moral problems.

Chapter 11

MAKING CONTACT AND
MAKING DECISIONS

Almost everything which has been and will be discussed implies contact between the patient and the professional. Whether it is a doctor, nurse, social worker, dentist, physiotherapist, or whoever, the focus of the whole process of decision-making is a face-to-face meeting. Whether this is called a meeting, an interview or a consultation does not matter; it is the time when two individuals meet and decisions are made. It may not matter whether or not the decision is right (though it undoubtedly helps if it is!) but if this part of the process is not properly conducted then all concerned can suffer. While many decisions affecting the patient may be discussed in case conferences or team meetings, as we shall bring out in Chapter 12, it is necessary that at some point there should be a one-to-one review of the situation, if for no other reason than to get the patient's views on the problem and the possible management. For convenience, we shall call this part of the decision-making process the 'consultation'.

Many issues of morality are raised by the consultation itself. Some of these will be covered in this chapter; others, such as consent and teamwork, will be discussed in more detail subsequently. This chapter will deal with the consultation process itself, discuss the management of uncertainty, then review some of the moral aspects, including telling the truth, confidentiality, paternalism, and the role of the professional.

1. THE CONSULTATION

The consultation is a highly complex process but is the focus of moral decision-making for individual patients. It is a process which is often quite frightening for the junior doctor or nurse, as, for perhaps the first time, they must respond to questions, think carefully about what they say, and be responsible for their actions. There may be no one around to give advice and help. Perhaps that is why so many shy away from the process.

A consultation occurs when a patient comes to a professional for advice about a problem, such as an illness or disease which is present or suspected. We shall identify and discuss to a varying extent seven morally relevant features of the consultation.

1. *Consent* is implied for at least some investigative procedures and treatment. Consent of this minimum kind is implied because the patient has voluntarily come for the consultation. We shall say more about consent in Chapter 18, and reference should also be made to the discussion of paternalism in section 4 of this chapter and to autonomy in Chapter 4, section 2.

2. *Confidentiality* is implied about the content of the interview. We shall discuss confidentiality in section 5 of this chapter.

3. The consultation requires that *communication and listening* should occur between the patient and the professional. This is a key feature of the consultation as it is the method by which problems are defined and solutions are discussed. Communication, however, is not a one-way process, it requires skills in listening both to the verbal and non-verbal messages given to professionals by patients. As was discussed in Chapter 2, the presenting problems of the patient may not be the only, the most important or even the real reason for the visit in the first place. Listening is a skill which is often underdeveloped in busy doctors and nurses. It is very easy to hear what you really want to hear, rather than what the patient is telling you. The other side of the coin is the ability of professionals to talk to patients about difficult and complex problems, about which there may be some

uncertainty, in language which is understandable to them, without being unnecessarily patronizing. This is not an easy task, and anyone who says it is has not been in the front line very often.

4. Another morally important feature of the consultation is *courtesy*. This, like many other things in this book, may seem to be only common sense. Yet how easy it is to forget. Remembering names, introducing yourself, explaining procedures, saying thank you, goodbye, and treating the individual opposite you with care and respect. Try the 'my mother' solution. If it was your mother across the table how would you wish her to be treated? In a busy ward or clinic, or during the rush of a home visit, it is easy to forget such simple things, yet they mean a great deal to individual patients. Remember how privileged you are to be party to the patients' problems and to be allowed to share in them. The health care professions are also vocations and doctors and nurses are *expected* by patients and the public at large to have commitment and compassion. They are expected to have a particular role as caring individuals. The concept of role has already been discussed, and we shall pick it up again later in this chapter.

5. Much of what has been discussed so far is related to the *quality of care* given. Professionals, after all, have had special training in their own particular fields, and the patient and public expect a certain quality and excellence from the care provided. When the quality goes down, patients' problems and anxieties begin to surface. (Chapter 19.)

6. This brings us to another relevant feature of the consultation − the development of *mutual trust and honesty*. Without mutual trust and honesty subsequent decisions, which may have important moral implications, will be less than satisfactory. We shall discuss truth-telling in section 3 of this chapter, but in the meantime we ask: If trust and honesty are essential in any relationship why not between a patient and a professional?

7. Finally, it is a very real privilege for the professional to be able to be part of the patient's life and to be told about his

problems. The word *compassion* was used in earlier chapters to describe the morally appropriate response to this privilege.

In this section the importance of seven morally relevant features of the consultation have been highlighted. They are: consent, confidentiality, communication and listening, courtesy, quality of care, mutual trust and honesty, and compassion. It will be taken as read that all professionals have some commitment to these ideals and concepts. In the sections that follow and in subsequent chapters these ideals will be developed, qualified, and sometimes challenged. One final aspect of the consultation should be mentioned, that of resource allocation. The consultation and the associated diagnosis and prognosis set out possible treatments and thus a commitment to resources. There are therefore important ethical issues associated with this part of the process and they will be discussed more fully in Chapter 17.

By way of a postscript to this section we shall discuss the role of the receptionist.

We have discussed in some detail the morally significant features of the consultation, assuming that this is the patient's first contact with health care on a given occasion. But there is an important qualification to be made here. The first contact may be with the receptionist or the secretary. For example, someone may feel unwell and may ring up, or a relative may ring up the GP. The first contact is then with whoever answers the telephone – receptionist, secretary, wife, or other relative. Now there are two well-known features of such initial contacts. The first is that the potential patient or his spokesman is, or is expected by the receptionist to be, demanding of attention for trivial ailments. The second is that the receptionist or spouse is very protective of the professional involved. The result can be that the initial contact with health care can be marred by abrupt or rude behaviour. The receptionist, in fact, will normally ask what is wrong and then make the decision as to whether a visit is required or as to how urgent the need for attention is. These decisions may be made without the doctor's knowledge.

A similar situation arises when patients arrive at an out-patient clinic. They will be anxious, confused, in unfamiliar surroundings, and so on. The attitudes and courtesy displayed at the reception desk are therefore important, especially since the patients may need to wait for attention.

It is also important to remember that the attitudes displayed by receptionists, porters, etc., will be influenced by the attitudes shown to them by the professional health care team or the individual doctor. If the receptionists are made to feel part of the health care team they will respond to patients with appropriate behaviour. These points will be discussed further in Chapter 12. It should be noted that many of the issues raised in this section relate to the Patients' Charter initiatives (see Chapter 20).

2. THE MANAGEMENT OF UNCERTAINTY

In almost all clinical decisions there is an element of uncertainty. Most biological phenomena have a normal value, around which the population of measurements is distributed – for instance pulse rate, temperature, and blood pressure. In terms of disease, illness and treatments there is once again a normal range and, on an individual basis, there will be variations from these norms. For example:

The normal postoperative period after appendicectomy is 3–5 days.
The normal period of time for recovery after a head cold is 2–3 days.
It will take, on average, 3 months to be fully rehabilitated after a hip replacement.
It will take 4–6 weeks to adjust to a colostomy, and to establish an appropriate diet and routine.

In all of these relatively simple facts there is variation between one individual and another. This becomes more complex when the question of success of treatment, or treatment complications, are included. For example:

Following appendicectomy there is a 5 per cent chance of developing a wound infection. The success rate, in non-small cell lung cancer, using chemotherapy as treatment, is less than 20 per cent as measured by objective response. Following mastectomy there is a 25 per cent incidence of psychological upset in the following year.

The point here is that though the information is available on a population basis, the information for the individual is uncertain. This important point was first introduced in Chapter 2. It follows that questions such as 'How long has he got to live?' are full of uncertainty.

Now, since the information which is available to the doctor or nurse is not certain, the way in which it is presented can be varied according to the value judgement of the professional. Take the incidence of wound infection after the removal of the appendix given above. This could be presented as:

(a) 'There is very little chance of your developing a wound infection and I'm sure you'll be home in five days.'
(b) 'We'll have to wait for a few days to see if the wound becomes infected; if so you might not go home in five days.'
(c) 'One in 20 patients gets a wound infection which keeps him in hospital longer than five days.'

It is a matter of value judgement which of these approaches (or many others) is adopted.

Patients and their families are looking for answers to specific questions, which are of major importance to them, yet the professional may not know the answer, or be able to give it only in terms of averages, ranges or probabilities. There are several ways to deal with this dilemma, and to manage the uncertainty.

1. *Say nothing.* This is a very useful way of dealing with the problem. It is also remarkably easy. The disadvantages must be very obvious; and the advantage, that at least false information would not be given, is hardly a strong one. But in some circumstances there may be merit in this approach.

2. *Make a clear and unequivocal statement.* This implies that you know the answer, are in full command of the situation and you personally never have patients who have wound infections –

the ward sister wouldn't allow it! Once again, this is a useful way of handling some areas of uncertainty. The difficulty is that something might go wrong and the course you have charted for the patient might need to change.

3. *Say you don't know the answer*. This is a very honest way of dealing with some areas of uncertainty. It does mean, however, that the patient has nothing to hold on to, no information on which to base decisions of his or her own. With this approach, the professional exposes his own weaknesses and vulnerability. It requires a great deal of self-confidence to adopt this approach, but it does have advantages in some instances.

4. *Take a middle road*. Say you can't be sure, give the probabilities or norms, and select an answer which you think, in your judgement, will apply. This approach may mean giving quite a lot of information to the patient − listing complications, problems, and options, and then selecting. During this your own weaknesses and indecisions may be exposed. It is, however, a useful method with some patients.

It should be apparent that the caricatures given above are not mutually exclusive and a doctor, nurse, or social worker may use all of them at any one time, with the same patient or with different ones. Look at these ways of dealing with uncertainty and, in the following case-histories, choose the one you think is most appropriate. Remember, no particular knowledge is assumed in answering these questions: assume that it is *you* the patient is asking, not the consultant or ward sister.

- A 46-year-old woman has just been admitted for removal of gallstones. This is a routine operation, with a low risk of post-operative complications (overall 5 per cent) and the usual time in hospital is 7 days. Her daughter's eighteenth birthday falls exactly on day seven after the operation. Before the operation she asks you whether she will be home in time.
  What is your reply?

- The wife of a 62-year-old man asks to see you. Her husband has lung cancer which has not responded well to treatment and

he now has rapidly progressive disease. Experience shows that survival at this stage is usually less than two months. She asks you how long he has to live.
What is your reply?

- A 38-year-old man has just had the diagnosis of multiple sclerosis made. This is a disease characterized by relapses and remissions which can progress at varying rates, but may be fatal in 2–20 years. This is his first episode, and he asks you about the prognosis.
What do you reply?

In your answers to these questions it is easy to say, 'Well, I don't have enough information' or 'I have no experience of that condition'. Yet in practical terms these are the kinds of question you may well be asked by patients and their families. If you *don't* know the answer to the question (which may well be the case) then presumably you could run away (which again may well be possible) or you can try to give an answer.

This section has tried to introduce the concept of uncertainty with clinical decision-making. When this is extended to include (as it must) the moral decisions which are required to be made, then the complexity of the problem is much increased. Read again Chapter 2, section 2, and read Chapter 14, section 2. We shall now look at a particular aspect of this problem of uncertainty, that is, telling the truth.

3. TELLING THE TRUTH

In our normal everyday contact with our family, friends and colleagues it is normal to tell the truth. Why then should it be any different with patients? The answer of course is that it shouldn't be, but before accepting this fully, ask yourself honestly in dealing with friends and family:

- Do you always tell the truth?
- Do you always tell the whole truth?
- Have you ever told lies?

● Has there ever been a 'good' reason for telling a lie?

Honest answers to these questions will probably reveal that in some circumstances the 'whole' truth is not told, and that occasionally it is possible to lie for a 'good' reason. Look again at Chapter 9, exercise 2.

Let us for the moment assume that 'telling the truth' is a good thing, and that in clinical practice this should be the normal procedure. Early in this book we divided knowledge into factual, practical and attitudinal, and it is useful to look at each of these in relation to 'telling the truth'.

The knowledge base: When patients ask questions about factual matters it is relatively simple to give answers. For example:

Your pulse rate is 76/min and regular.
Your blood pressure is 120/80, that is normal.
The pain is related to gallstones.
The enlarged lymph nodes in your neck are malignant.

These facts are fairly straightforward and could be readily communicated to the patient.

● In the examples given above, are there any which you would *not* wish to communicate, given that the answers are correct, and that the patient has asked the question?

The answer is more complex when a wide range of information is available. Take a patient with lung cancer. A series of investigations, and clinical examinations show that:

the histology is non-small cell lung cancer;
it affects the left lower lobe of the lung;
there is infection of the lung, distal to the tumour;
there is hilar enlargement indicating lymph node involvement;
the right lung is clear;
liver function tests and liver ultrasound show metastases;
there are several skin nodules which are malignant;
a bone scan shows several suspicious areas in the lumbar spine;
a CT scan of brain is normal.

The details above are presented in technical language. In answering questions these would be discussed using appropriate words.

- Before proceeding to the question below try to translate each of these terms into ordinary language.
- The patient (his wife, with whom you have built up a good relationship, is present) asks:
  'I know I have lung cancer, but has it spread?'
  What would you reply to this? Would you give all of the above information, or would you withhold some of it?

Practical knowledge: This deals with the skills required and the possible outcome of treatment. The uncertainty which can occur here has already been raised, and is a real and practical problem. This is particularly the case with possible results of treatment, and prognosis, where uncertainty may be very great indeed.

Questions of moral attitudes: This is concerned with your attitudes as to whether patients should, or should not be told the truth. There are several aspects to this.

1. Are there circumstances when you would *not* tell the truth?
2. Are there circumstances when you would tell a lie?
3. Are there circumstances when you would not tell the *whole* truth?
4. Are there circumstances when you would *force* the truth on a patient − when you would confront him with the truth for his own good?

- Think about these four groups of circumstances and ask yourself whether or not you feel that such approaches are *ever* justified. Give examples if you can.

Coping strategies: Throughout this decision it has been assumed that patients and their families wish to know the truth, as this will help them to deal with the illness and to cope more effectively with the problems. This is an important assumption as it in turn makes assumptions about how people deal with problems and uncertainty. There is a range of strategies which can be used by individuals. What is important to note is that these strategies may be used by the *same* people but at *different* times in their illness. For this reason the *communication strategy* adopted may also be different. Among the range of strategies which are available to individuals here are some of the most common.

1. *Acceptance*: The patient and family accept the diagnosis and its implications. They wish to get on with treatment and ask few questions.

2. *Denial*: The patient denies that there is an illness, or that the illness is serious. Information can be given but will not be absorbed. 'The doctor won't tell me what's wrong' is a common response at this stage.

3. *Knowledgeable involvement*: The patient wishes as much information as possible and wants to be kept fully in the picture. He, or she, intends to fight the illness by dealing with it logically and analytically. Typically these patients ask lots of questions.

4. *Anxiety, fear, and confusion*: The patient and the family are overwhelmed by the enormity of the diagnosis and its implications. They do not know where to go for advice.

5. *Anger and frustration*: The patient and family are angry, often with the health care team, and are frustrated that they cannot do anything about the problem.

Once again these are 'cameos' and several other strategies or combinations of strategy can be used by patients to deal with their problems. The question for this section is: How do you communicate the 'truth' to such patients in the various different categories? Look at this example.

● Following a period of generally feeling unwell, an 8-year-old boy is given a blood test which results in the diagnosis of acute leukaemia. He is the oldest child of three and the parents were told the diagnosis two days ago by the general practitioner. He gave them a general and fairly optimistic picture of the future, but they (the parents and son) are coming to see you about future management. You will be able to tell them that with treatment there is a 70 per cent chance of cure. The treatment will involve a 6-month course of chemotherapy, with radio-therapy, and that there will be the possibility of serious side-effects. These would include infection, haematological problems, and alopecia.

What would you say to the parents who, in your assessment, were in one of the following coping states?

Acceptance
Denial
Knowledgeable involvement
Anxiety-fear-confusion
Anger and frustration.

Would what you say differ in each of these categories?

This section has tried to emphasize the importance of telling the truth, but also to highlight the difficulties. Three further factors will now be emphasized.

1. The importance of listening to patients: this cannot be emphasized too strongly.
2. The importance of time: it takes time for the implications of diagnosis to sink in. It takes time to give information, and information may need to be given over a period of time.
3. The importance of choice: telling the truth allows the patient to have some choice in his management.

A quotation from St Bernard might be an appropriate way of ending this section, 'Bitter is truth unseasoned by grace'.

4. PATERNALISM

A discussion of communication and truth-telling takes us naturally into the subject of paternalism. Paternalism is not the exclusive province of male doctors, but 'maternalism' has other connotations so we shall use 'paternalism' for the attitude which both males and females can display. Paternalism is the protection of individuals from self-inflicted harm, in the way that a father or mother looks after children. Decisions are taken, choices made and freedom inhibited, all for the good of the patient. There is no element of consent. In this sense paternalism is not 'bad' in its intentions.

Paternalism can manifest itself in three basic ways: in language, in behavioral and in decision-making. Take language, and look at these examples:

'We're going to give you treatment today.'
'Now then, my dear.'
'Aren't we looking well today.'
'Have you been a good patient?'
'If you're very good we'll let you home on Saturday.'

As far as behaviour is concerned it is easy to find examples of paternalistic activity. For example:

Standing above patients.
Keeping them waiting.
Being condescending.

Above all, paternalism is shown in the taking of decisions for others which they have a right to take for themselves.

'It would not do you any good if you knew.'
'Let me make the decisions.'
'You don't need to know.'

Some of what is objectionable in paternalism relates to a lack of *courtesy*, but above all it is an offence against *autonomy*.

Read Chapter 4, section 2, and then

● List the advantages and disadvantages of paternalism as you see them.

5. CONFIDENTIALITY

The consultation, or interview, between the patient and the professional requires the development of trust, as we said in section 1. This is built up by proper two-way communication, a central feature of which is confidentiality. It is implicit in this relationship that whatever is divulged remains confidential. This has been part of medical practice since the time of the Hippocratic Oath. Clinical practice is concerned with dealing with whole patients, not just the physical problems, but with social, psychological, emotional, and spiritual problems. To do this effectively, however, requires that a team approach is adopted, and that there is communication between members of the team. This raises the fundamental problem of confidentiality in the health care professions: How do you share confidential information without losing trust?

This problem, of course, is not exclusively a medical one. Nurses, social workers, dietitians, and physiotherapists all face the same dilemma. Information is given in confidence, and the question is how much of it should be shared.

Levels of information: It is possible to identify a series of levels of information, which might be used to decide on whether or not the information could be shared. There are four levels. Look at each one carefully and ask whether this information could be divulged within the team.

Identification: Name, address, sex, marital status, and primary disease.

Medical information: Disease, extent of disease, treatment investigations, past medical information, drug information.

Social information: Housing, work, family, social relationships.

Psychological information: Anxiety, stress, sexual problems, emotional state.

At present this information is stored, presented, and shared in a variety of ways:

Documents, reports, case-sheets, nursing Kardex, etc.
Tutorials, or formal doctor−doctor, nurse−nurse contact.
Ward meetings, formal or informal, where problems are shared and discussed.
Ward rounds, with discussion between the staff.

Letters giving information are exchanged between staff. Investigation forms are completed and sent throughout the hospital, and into the community.

In the process of sharing this information two assumptions are made:

1. The patient has agreed to this sharing.
2. The information remains confidential within the team. A typical team on a medical or surgical ward would include doctors, nurses, social workers, physiotherapists, dietitians, pharmacists, and others. Related to this team are secretaries, receptionists, porters, and ward maids. These individuals are vital to the working of the team.

As an exercise read the following clinical profile and try to answer the questions at the end. The profile has been arbitrarily divided into the four levels of information given above.

1. Mrs Irene McGregor is a 55-year-old married woman who lives on a housing estate in the suburbs of a large city. She has been admitted for a hysterectomy related to fibroids.

2. Routine chest radiograph shows evidence of previous tuberculosis. Other investigations are normal. In the past she has had no serious illness, but 10 years ago was investigated for possible epilepsy.

3. She has three children, all of whom are well, but one has recently been suspected of drug-taking. She has told this only to the social worker. Her husband is a postman and she works part-time in a shop. There is an elderly mother-in-law who lives near by and is visited daily by the family.

4. She is naturally anxious about the operation, and the fact that her eldest son may be involved with drugs has made her particularly anxious about the admission. She is otherwise well adjusted although, because of her symptoms, normal sexual relationships with her husband have been difficult. She is quite concerned about this.

- This information, except for that associated with her son, has been obtained from the case-sheet. Who should have access to it?
- How much of each of the four levels of information should be shared with members of the professional staff?
- How much should be shared with other members of the team, porters, receptionists, etc.?
- Do all members of staff need to know all the information?
- During the weekly ward meeting, a member of the nursing staff feels that the patient is more anxious than she should be. How much information about the son should be divulged and openly discussed?

While answering these questions have you formed any views on the rules for maintaining confidentiality?

It is sometimes useful, when deciding on who should be given confidential information, to separate people into the following groups:

(1) those who must know;
(2) those who should know;
(3) those who could know;
(4) those who shouldn't know.

Look again at Mrs McGregor and the issues and questions which have been raised. Divide the professional groups, the supporting staff, and others into the categories listed above.

Confidentiality, outside the health care team: So far it has been assumed that information about an individual *might* be shared between members of the team. There are circumstances, however, when information about a particular patient is requested by other groups. Consider Mrs McGregor again. Information is requested by the following. Would you divulge it?

- The husband: He asks for information about the medical problems.

- A close friend: A neighbour (female) asks to see the ward sister and requests information about treatment.

- The social services: They are concerned about possible problems at home while the patient is recovering. They wish details of the family background.

- The police: Questions are being asked about possible drug problems in the area and they suspect her son.

- The press: They have found out from the police that her son is a possible addict. They phone you for information.

- Your colleagues: You meet a colleague at a social event. He (or she) is very interested in family problems associated with drug-taking. He asks if you know anyone who might help in this important research project.

These points raise important issues in confidentiality, and you should now be clearer about when, and to whom, you would divulge information.

Computers and records: The introduction of computers and databases has introduced a new element into the maintenance of confidentiality. It has always been possible (but rather difficult) to obtain access to case-sheets, the Data Protection act makes this clear. The introduction of records and data on computer files follows the provision in the Act and allows for patients to have access to these also. So much is clear, though there are still some fundamental moral questions which need to be discussed.

- Will this prevent the writing down of sensitive information?

- Who else will have access to the information? Should relatives be allowed to see it?

- The first principle of the Act relates to 'fair obtaining'. That is, that the information gained must be for a specific purpose, and cannot, except by consent, be used for other purposes. Can you think of situations in which data which has been legitimately obtained for clinical purposes might then be used for other reasons?

6. THE ROLE OF THE PROFESSIONAL

In this discussion about making contact and making decisions it has been assumed that the health care professional has a particular role in this process. However, as was discussed in Chapter 6, professional roles may vary from time to time, and indeed professional, public, and individual roles may merge. The doctor, for example, may act as a healer, a technician, a counsellor, an educator, or a friend, or indeed many other roles. The following list gives an idea of the wide variety of roles that *any* health care professional might adopt.

Healer: The primary function here is one of caring and healing. All professional health care groups have this as a basic function.

Technician: There is a technical role in almost all professional activities, whether it is in performing an operation, dressing a wound, massaging a leg, pulling a tooth, or knowing the relevant section of welfare legislation.

Counsellor: Much of the routine work of health care workers is dealing with the psychological and social problems of patients and their families. In some instances this may even overlap with the spiritual area.

Educator: Teaching is an important role of those who work in the health services. This may involve professional, public, or patient education.

Scientist: Most groups have a responsibility to develop new ideas and to investigate the causes and treatment of disease.

Friend: In some areas of clinical practice it is not difficult to become friends with the patient and the family. In some instances this may mean that the professional role, for example as a healer, may conflict with the role as a friend.

Political: Doctors, nurses and other health care workers, because of their special knowledge, may, because they feel strongly about it, become involved in political activities. Campaigns against cigarette smoking, drugs, or alcohol abuse, nuclear power, are obvious areas of involvement.

Private: Health care workers are also private citizens with their own feelings and beliefs. There is considerable pressure, from many sources, to make them conform to certain ideals. In dress and behaviour, for example, doctors and nurses are expected to live up to certain values, and in some instances to set examples for the public.

These, then, are some of the roles which can be adopted by health care workers. There may be many more. Look again at the case of Mrs Irene McGregor, the lady who has been admitted for a hysterectomy. She asks you a series of questions which you are expected to answer. Once again forget about the level of knowledge that you may one day have; answer the questions as you are now. Would you see your role changing as you answer these questions?

- Tell me what happens when I have a hysterectomy?
- What does a shadow on my chest radiograph mean?
- What will I do about my son?
- Can I get some help with my mother-in-law?
- What causes fibroids?
- I don't seem to be getting on well with my husband. What should I do?
- Why don't you *do* something about the drug problem?

The concept of role is a useful one in enabling us to see the various ways in which we can respond to problems, and questions from patients. It is limited, however, in that it does not highlight the very individual talents of each professional. But it should make us more aware of how easy it becomes to slip into a 'professional' role while dealing with patients. Read Chapter 6, sections 3 and 4.

7. CONCLUSION

This chapter has dealt with a series of topics related to making contact with patients and making decisions. The key topic is the development of a range of moral features in the patient—professional relationship. In discussing these we put in a practical context concepts such as trust, truth-telling, confidentiality, and paternalism. The major difficulty is in the handling of uncertainty.

Chapter 12

WORKING TOGETHER

Teams are common in many walks of life − in business, sport, and industry − and in the health care professions which deal with patients or clients teamwork is also important. To pay lip-service to the concept, however, is not to say that working together is easy, nor that it happens everywhere. Nevertheless, teamwork is an integral part of the work of the health care professional, whether the team is in an operating theatre, a geriatric ward, or in primary health care.

In health service some teams are small and some are large, but they are all based on the same principles. Before looking at some of the moral problems posed by working in teams it is necessary to look at some of these principles, which govern the ways in which teams are organized and function. As these principles are outlined, look closely at them and try to analyse for yourself whether or not such principles are justifiable, and indeed whether teams are necessary. Some aspects of teamwork, such as confidentiality, have already been discussed. Read Chapters 6 and 7, and Chapter 11, section 5.

1. THE BASIS OF TEAMWORK

Teams are always governed by a set of principles or assumptions, although these are not always made explicit. We shall deal with four:

1. *Teams have common aims or goals*. This may seem self-evident, and it is increasingly common for a team in a health care setting to state clearly what are its specific goals. The goals may be broadly defined: 'to do the best for the patient', 'to care for the community' or some such phrase. Nevertheless, unless goals are openly discussed as some form of 'mission statement' then some members of the team may not be clear as to the overall purposes of the team. This can lead to conflict, where different professionals have different goals.

● Think of your current position in the hospital or the community. Ask yourself if the aims of the team with which you are working are well-defined. If you are a student, think about the clinical unit to which you are attached at present. Does it have a team? What are the aims of the team that you can observe?

2. *Each member of the team has a distinctive and important role* and the effectiveness of the team would be diminished without each member. The role of each member is clear. Now, while such an idealistic assumption may be considered the best one to adopt, some questions must be asked. For example:

● Are all members of the team really equal?
● Are all members of the team really necessary?
● Are roles fixed or are they interchangeable?

This latter question bears closer examination. Take the following situation:

A 65-year-old man, who two months ago had a stroke, has returned to the hospital for a follow-up visit. He has made good progress, is now mobile, but still has a slight speech defect. During his initial admission he was noted to be hypertensive and was started on drug treatment for this, and was put on a weight-reducing diet. He asks the following questions:

Will my treatment be changed today?
Do I need to continue with my speech therapy and physiotherapy?
Can I have a home help?

Should I continue with my diet?

Try to answer these questions from the point of view of being a doctor, a nurse, a social worker, a physiotherapist, a dietitian, and a speech therapist. How far are the roles of each interchangeable? Can each of the professionals listed answer all of the questions? Should they be able to?

Working in teams means being able to recognize one's own limitations, and the strengths of others. Too strict a definition of roles, however, may set limitations for the team. Sometimes a centre-forward has to play full-back. It is necessary, however, if teams are to function properly, that members are able to practise together, become aware of each other's strengths and weaknesses, and share problems.

3. *Most teams have leaders*, so why should not those dealing with patients? This is one of the most contentious issues in health care practice. Most would agree that someone has to make the final decision about the patient, but who? Most would also agree that, without leadership, direction and purpose can be lost, and that committee decisions are not always the most satisfactory for the patient or for the team. There can be delays in reaching decisions. An effective leader has several functions:

First-hand knowledge and experience of the particular health care area.
The ability to identify the tasks to be done, and to be able to get them done.
To help the team work together and to look after its members.
To ensure that each member of the team plays his or her part to the full.

Such a list of functions of a leader can, of course, be disputed and discussed and it is hoped that they will provide a basis for this. If for the moment they can be accepted, the important question is whether or not they identify a particular professional group as being the 'leaders', or whether all professional groups could provide this function.

Think again of the patient described earlier, the man with the stroke who has returned for a follow-up visit. It is quite possible that all professionals could have answered all of the questions. But who should be the leader and make the final decisions on future policy, including the patient's after-care in the community? (For the moment let us assume that the patient is also involved. We shall discuss this in more detail later.)

The situation is often complicated by the fact that patients may be being cared for by several different clinical groupings. For example, a patient may initially be referred to a physician, who then refers to a surgeon, who then refers to a radiotherapist. Including the primary care team, there are now four groups involved. Thus, in addition to interprofessional teamwork (between doctors, nurses, social workers, etc.), there must also be teamwork between the different clinical units. Without this it is undoubtedly the patient who suffers.

4. *Teams are able to measure their performance.* In sporting terms a team would be seen to be ineffective if it did not win the occasional game. League tables provide a measure of such performance. People want to belong to a 'good' team and to support it. But what of the health care situation? How is it possible to measure the performance? In Chapter 17 we discuss several ways in which this could be accomplished and costed. Within a small group, such as a ward team, or a primary health care team, one way is to carry out a regular audit of the work of the unit. This can be in relation to a particular topic, such as referrals to a specialist service, out-patient services, etc., or to the overall results of a particular treatment or service. In this way there is regular feedback on the outcome. It follows that there will be times when it will be known that performance is poor and the service needs to be changed. This is always a challenge to the team and to its leadership.

5. *The structure and stability of health care teams.* In the above discussion it has been assumed that teams, whatever their size or special interest, are relatively stable. Consider a team in a general surgical unit. It might be composed of:

consultant surgeon   student nurse
ward sister   social worker

specialist in training	physiotherapist
staff nurse	dietitian
house officer	health visitor

- How long will each be a member of the team? For example, the house officer or student nurse will be a member for several months only.
- What implication does a rapidly changing staff have for the functions of the team?
- What implications does it have for team leadership?

Teams therefore, in general, have a common purpose, and each member of the team has a particular role. Within the team, however, there should be the facility for changing roles. Teams normally have leaders, but it is an open question as to who this should be. Teams measure their performance in order to improve the level of care provided. With these basis assumptions in mind let us now look at some of the *moral* problems of working in teams.

2. MORAL PROBLEMS OF WORKING IN TEAMS

Many of these arise from differences in values between individuals. This is not entirely surprising. If you brought together ten people to work on a complicated problem which has moral implications then it would be strange if differences of opinion did not emerge. It is important to remember this, as differences in opinion may be based more on individual views than on the party professional line. Some of the problems of working in teams have already been discussed. Communication, confidentiality, truth-telling, and patient rights are just some of the issues which will be developed further in this chapter.

A particular problem is that of conflict between health care professionals. This can arise for many reasons and can involve intra- and interprofessional differences. An important question for all, therefore, is how to deal with such conflict. This issue will be taken up at the end of this chapter. However, during the following section consider carefully the implications of *not* agreeing with your colleagues. What would, or should, your attitude be to differences of opinion? No matter what professional group you belong to such differences will arise in the course of your work, and you may have to be ready to deal with them. (Read Chapter 7, section 2.)

3. COMMUNICATION PROBLEMS

This is a particularly common type of problem. One member of the team has made a decision, perhaps even discussed it with the patient, but has not communicated it to the rest of the team. Often it is the junior nurse or doctor who is faced with the patient who asks the awkward or leading question. Unless each member of the team is involved then how can responses be appropriate?

The discussion so far has assumed that a decision has been made but not communicated within the team. There is, however, the other side of the coin − sometimes no decision has been made. Once again, confronted by a patient, what does the doctor or nurse do if a question is asked? This is a special problem when it has been decided (for good or ill) that a patient should not be told of the diagnosis. It may be that others in the team feel that this is not the way to proceed and wish the patient to be informed.

- Who has the final authority in this instance? What would you do if you disagreed?

The question of course can be broadened to include management and treatment decisions. What if you do not agree with the decisions made? To whom would you complain? (Read Chapter 7, section 1.)

These problems argue for clear lines of communication between members of the team. But how can this best be achieved?

- Consider how you could improve communication in your clinical area. If you are not yet a full member of one team, how would you organize the channels of communication

(1) within your own professional group?
(2) with others in the team?

4. TREATMENT AND RESEARCH POLICIES

Many clinical teams have evolved treatment policies and procedures over the years. the medical and nursing staff have become familiar and comfortable with them. There is a stable routine which everyone understands. Into this put a new practice, procedure or research project. It does not much matter whether this is a medical or nursing change, it is likely to upset the balance. There are two problems to be considered. The first is how the team reacts to the change and deals with the innovation. If these matters are not handled properly, then the conflict can spread to other aspects of work, and patient care can suffer. The new procedure, for example, could take up more time or resources and some might feel that this could affect the service provided. The second aspect is whether or not there are moral objections to the new procedure. This is particularly the case with research projects which may disrupt the routine or may even be considered to be morally wrong by individual members of the team. The use of experimental drugs which can have side-effects is one example; or some members of the team may have very strong objections to taking part in abortions. In these circumstances, where there is a very strong objection to the practice, the individual must have the right to opt out.

It could be argued, however, that this means that others have to do the work, and that those opting out are simply abrogating their responsibility to the patient and to the team. Consider the following:

● Suppose that a new procedure is to be introduced into the clinical unit, and one member of the team refuses on moral grounds to have anything to do with the work. How should the rest of the team react:

  Allow the individual to opt out?
  Make him do more of other work to compensate?

Ask him to leave?
Tell him to do it?

There may well be other ways of dealing with this problem which you can think of yourself. (Read Chapter 7.)

5. CONFIDENTIALITY

Working within a team means that information will be shared. Implicit in this is that such information is confidential. This topic was discussed in Chapter 11, section 5, but here we shall be concerned with the subject as it applied to teams. Within a closely-knit team there should be little problem with confidentiality, but as the team expands problems can arise. For example, do you consider that secretarial staff should have access to confidential information? It is highly likely that they do, and you must consider the safeguards you would adopt when this is the case.

● What safeguards would you suggest?

● What about those who are not part of the formal team but who might have a role in care? For example, does the minister or the priest have a right to be part of the team and to share the information? What about friends and lay helpers, members of support groups, or participation groups? How much should be shared, and how can confidentiality be preserved? These may seem like theoretical questions but it is remarkable how rapidly very confidential information travels in the hospital and the community.

6. THE PATIENT AS PART OF THE TEAM

In the discussions so far we have not considered whether patients should be part of the team and take a full part in the discussions. This question is slightly different from that of truth-telling, in that the patient might be involved, and indeed be part of the decision-making process, without necessarily having all the information available. It does, however, imply that the patient has a right to be part of the team. There are obviously advantages and disadvantages to this, from a practical and from a moral point of view.

• Do you think that patients should be part of the team in all circumstances, or are there times when they should be excluded?

The relatives often have a great deal to offer in the care of the patient. Nursing care, for example, can be a very rewarding way of involving the relatives, but they are often excluded, and not encouraged to be part of the caring team. At a moral level why should they be excluded at the very time when husbands and wives, parents, and children should be close? How would you feel if a child of yours was ill and you were barred from being part of the team? Do parents and spouses not also have rights?

7. DIFFERENCES IN GOALS

There is often the assumption that the team shares the same goals. In a general sense this is normally the case. But within the team differences can arise. Take our 65-year-old patient recovering from a stroke. Several goals are possible:

control of hypertension;
mobilization of the patient;
reduction of weight;
keeping him at home.

Consider the most important goal if you were a nurse, physiotherapist, dietitian, or doctor. Would they be different? If so, could this result in problems within the team? Suppose, for example, that the blood pressure was not well controlled, and that the medical staff decide to admit the patient to hospital for further treatment. This might well conflict with the objectives of the social work staff who wish if at all possible to keep the patient at home. The primary care team are also likely to resent this, and could also see it as a failure of their team. What could therefore be seen as a fairly straightforward decision to admit a patient, could be seen to diminish the importance of the goals of some professional groups.

8. GENERAL MANAGEMENT AND CLINICAL TEAMS

The introduction of general management and the National Health Service reforms have focused attention much more on value for money and the use of resources. The clinical team will have an important input into both the purchasing of health care and its provision. The maintenance of proper standards will be of concern to professionals. Thus, the implications of changing the pattern of care by altering the location of a clinical service, for example, or closing a hospital or ward, inevitably raise issues for health care staff. This can bring the professional into the public or even the political arena. There are mechanisms in place to ensure that there is adequate opportunity for discussions with management. In consequence, 'whistle-blowing' ought not to be undertaken without careful consideration.

• Are there issues about which you might feel sufficiently strongly to take such action?

9. COMPLEMENTARY MEDICINE

There is increasing public and professional awareness of the potential of techniques which are not ordinarily available in the Health Service. Such methods, sometimes called 'alternative' therapies, include hypnosis, acupuncture, herbal remedies, biofeedback techniques, the Alexander technique, visualization, spiritual healing, etc. It is often said that even if such techniques do no good, at least they do no harm. There is some evidence that this may not be entirely true and that some methods can be harmful, although some may succeed where orthodox medicine has failed. The question at issue here, however, is whether or not those who practise such techniques should be part of the team.

Take the 59-year-old woman with severe rheumatoid arthritis who comes to the surgery for a routine visit. During the conversation she says that she wishes to go to a faith healer.

● How do you react to that? What advice would you give her? Would you encourage her to go?

Suppose that she wishes to try some other form of alternative therapy. Do you have a view on which therapies you would support and which you would not? One concern of patients who do try such techniques is that their ordinary medical and nursing advisers will be cross at the thought that their treatment is clearly not sufficient and that perhaps the patient will not be welcomed back.

● How do you react to that suggestion?

A final and very important question is why patients go for alternative therapy in the first place. Several reasons can be found, including dissatisfaction with current medical and nursing practice and the way in which individual patients are handled.

● Can you think of reasons why patients choose alternative therapies? If these are partly related to the health care system, what would you do about it?

10. SUPPORT WITHIN THE TEAM

One of the important functions of the team is that it provides support for all who are part of the team. This is sometimes called the 'therapeutic community'. There is a system of help and problems are shared. This can be done in a variety of ways including formal sessions with a counsellor or psychiatrist. It can be done informally by the leaders of the team listening to members of staff and by making themselves accessible to those who need help. Social occasions are a very useful way of bringing the team together and allowing problems to surface.

Under most circumstances the identification of problems is a positive action. Individuals can be helped and perhaps given greater insight into the job.

Moral problems can arise, however, in relation to staff counselling. Suppose, for example, that it becomes apparent that one of the nurses in a renal unit is having problems in dealing with this group of patients. She is absent at times and while she is there does not really pull her weight. The other staff make up for this but are rather resentful. People begin to talk about her and even the patients begin to realise that something is wrong. The morale of the team is suffering and you have the moral problem in front of you to deal with. What would you do?

A different problem arises where a member of staff just does not fit in. In a hospice, for example, a junior doctor is appointed for a six-month rotational period. Shortly after he arrives it becomes clear that he is temperamentally unsuited to this kind of work. He is rude to patients, does not ask for help and does not keep other members of the team informed of his actions. The carefully built up esprit of the team is quickly destroyed and the atmosphere in the hospice changes. Patient care begins to suffer. What action would you take? (Read Chapter 7, section 2.)

A further example is that of illness among staff. Although the team will share some problems it is right to ask the question as to whether illness is a confidential matter. Obviously this depends on the problem, but the key question is what the team should do about it. This is sometimes called the 'sick doctor' or 'sick nurse' problem. The individual is clearly not functioning and other members of staff make up for this. In some instances the individual may even be a hazard to patients. Under these circumstances you might consider that you had a moral obligation to do something about it. In the case of the 'sick doctor' problem there is now a well worked out plan for identification of individuals at risk and help is available.

Perhaps the most important aspect of the therapeutic community is that all concerned recognize that at times there will be problems and that is the responsibility of the team to identify them and to share them. Such problems often occur in special teams which deal with very ill patients, where the stress level is very high. Under these circumstances individuals become very vulnerable and the 'burn-out' syndrome, where the doctor or nurse becomes emotionally and physically exhausted, is not uncommon.

11. QUESTIONING PARTICIPATION IN MEDICAL PROCEDURES

Much of the discussion above has been of a general nature. To focus the issues, it is useful to look specifically at the problems which arise if a member of the team disagrees with the decision or action of another member. Several nursing bodies have recently reviewed this issue and the following summarizes some of the arguments and possible actions of the nurse who disagrees with a doctor's decision.

Nurses, as part of their caring role, participate in medically prescribed treatment and procedures which it is the proper function of the medical practitioner to determine. The nurse is expected to co-operate with others involved in the care of the patient and mutual trust can be maintained only if that principle is observed. This may, however, conflict with the principle that the nurse must perform her duties in such a way as to prevent any avoidable harm to the patient.

If there were an objection to a procedure's being carried out it could be directed either at the procedure itself or more commonly at its being carried out in a given case. Abortion, or 'nursing care only' for certain neonates with Down's syndrome are examples of procedures where there might be objections to the treatment *per se*. Objections to the use of procedures in given cases are often based on the following allegations that:

1. There is a considerable risk of harm occurring.
2. Any possible benefits are small.
3. The patient does not consent to the procedure.

It is right that the nurse should question procedures, and that as a first priority the justification for a given procedure should be established. This should be done in a way which does not necessarily interfere with the treatment, or in any way hinder patient care. These matters are not to be solved by following set rules, but guide-lines can be useful in assisting the nurse to pursue her objection. These guide-lines might also be useful for other professions, and indeed for intraprofessional disagreements.

1. Seek clarification from the person who issued the instructions. Make sure that the factual basis of the objection is clear and that there is good documentation in the records and assessments of the procedure followed.
2. Discuss the matter with other nurses, at the same level, and if there is no satisfactory outcome, raise the matter at a higher level. A forum for the discussion of such matters might be useful.
3. Whenever possible the individuals who disagree should be brought together to try to resolve the question. In this instance clearly laid out written information may be helpful.
4. If none of these methods is satisfactory then a formal objection should be made, first making this known to the senior nurse and doctor involved.

For the student nurse the problems are different, in that the student cannot choose which areas of nursing practice she wishes to be involved in. Refusal of a student to take part would be justified only under the conditions listed above. Where a particular procedure upsets a nurse in training then guidance as to the future career should be given. (Read Chapter 7, section 1.)

12. TEACHING AND LEARNING IN TEAMS

An important function of all teams is that of teaching and learning. Each situation, each problem, each patient becomes a learning situation. As we discussed earlier in this book, the teaching of facts and information is usually carried out by someone of seniority, who has special knowledge of the subject.

While experience matters a great deal in dealing with moral problems, we also pointed out that everyone has values and that even the most junior member of the team may have a valid point of view to share with others. Indeed, such views may be new, refreshing, and stimulating. There are two aspects of this to be considered. The first concerns the junior member of staff who feels that he or she has a comment to make which may contribute to the decision. How is it possible to make the view heard? In this situation there is a responsibility on the junior member of staff to speak up and a responsibility on the seniors to listen. The second aspect is related to the learning value of such views for the rest of the team. The team must be open enough to listen and learn from all members of the team.

- Would you be prepared to learn from the experiences of another medical student or student nurse?

- Do you think consultants, ward sisters and senior social workers would?

13. DEALING WITH CONFLICT IN TEAMS

In everyday clinical practice in all specialties, there will be differences of opinion. In most cases these will be insignificant and of no real importance to you. Someone has made a decision with which you do not agree but, because he is more senior, you are prepared to stand by the decision and to take part in the subsequent action. Suppose, however, that a decision is made with which you disagree so passionately that you are not prepared to be party to it. Indeed, you may feel so strongly about it that you are even prepared to 'go public' and report the incident. To go to such extremes is very rare, but occasionally decisions or incidents are so morally repugnant that you might be prepared to make a stand. The problem may be within your own professional group or with a member of another profession. (Read Chapter 7, section 1).

- At this stage can you think of any situations where you might feel that you could be put in this position?

- If you do get to this stage there are several avenues open to you. Look at the following list (and you might be able to add more options) and consider what you would do.

    Ignore the problem, turn a blind eye.
    Raise it at the next team meeting.
    Raise it with management.
    Confront the individual and give your views.
    Write an anonymous letter.
    Speak to the person immediately senior to you.
    Resign.
    Make the affair public.

Such moral dilemmas are not confined to health care practice.

Prima donnas: Every professional group has its prima donnas – individuals who are specially gifted and with particular talents. Such individuals are often a law unto themselves, but because of their outstanding achievements their 'habits' are often tolerated. Most teams cannot tolerate prima donnas without either acquiescing in their every foible, or making them team leaders.

- Can you think, in your own experience, of special individuals who have dominated a clinical team?

- Should this be allowed?

14. CONCLUSION: ARE TEAMS WORTHWHILE?

So far the assumption has been made that teams have value. You may feel that the many points raised in this section of the book question that assumption. As a final exercise in this chapter, list the advantages and disadvantages of working together and come to your own conclusion as to the worth of teams.

Chapter 13
A QUESTION OF LIVING

When facing some problems of morality it can be helpful to reflect on the accumulated wisdom of mankind as expressed in moral rules and traditional pieces of advice. But this approach is of very little help when we are considering the range of possibilities which have arisen with the new technology relating to conception and contraception. There can be no traditional advice on this since it is only recently that the technology has existed, and indeed it is developing every year. But although there are no traditional answers let us hope that traditional arguments and approaches can still clarify our problems.

Discussion of infertility and its alleviation must centre on the Report of the Warnock Committee (1985) which reviews the best available evidence, discusses the legal and moral implications of the various techniques for alleviating infertility and makes recommendations for future discussion and possible legislation. Some of these recommendations are especially important in view of the shortage of babies for adoption.

1. ARTIFICIAL INSEMINATION

One of the techniques is that of artificial insemination, a technique which has been known for a long time in the veterinary context. It has been used more recently to help couples in two sorts of situation. First, there is the case where the man is not completely infertile. In this circumstance the semen may be concentrated and inserted directly into the uterus. The only arguments against this apparently useful extension of treatment for infertility are that it separates the unitive and the procreative functions of sexual intercourse, and that it involves masturbation, which some consider to be wrong. We do not regard these as strong arguments against this kind of treatment (AIH). The second technique, of artificial insemination by donor (AID), is more controversial. In this technique the semen comes from a donor other than the husband (because the husband or partner is effectively infertile) and is inserted into the wife's uterus. Apart from the weak arguments against AIH already mentioned, there are two arguments which apply to AID in particular. The first is that the introduction of a third party (the donor) into the marital relationship is wrong, and the second is that the effect on the child so conceived will be bad.

In assessing these arguments we must distinguish the view that the practice is wrong in itself from the view that it is wrong because of the consequences it will have on the marriage or the child. To see it as wrong in itself is to see it as a kind of adultery. But this does not seem a fair description, if we remember that it is a practice carried out with the consent of all parties, in a clinical context, with the identity of the donor kept secret, and above all without sexual intercourse between parties.

The second view, that it is wrong because of its effect on the marriage or the child, depends on empirical considerations. As far as the marriage is concerned, the couple involved embark on the treatment only when they have exhausted all other methods, and then only after counselling. Remaining childless is just as likely to have a deleterious effect on the marriage. As far as the child is concerned, she may well wish to know in due course the identity of her genetic father. But the fact that such information could become available might have an adverse effect on the recruitment of donors. At the moment this is just speculative.

AIH and especially AID raise moral problems but, on the whole, especially if the law on AID is altered, they seem reasonable extensions of infertility services.

- If you were interviewing a married couple for AID what questions would you ask?

- Would your attitude differ if the couple were unmarried?
- Would your attitude differ if the couple were lesbian?
- What would your attitude be to revealing the name of the donor to the child?
- Should this remain confidential?

2. *IN VITRO* FERTILIZATION

A new technique for alleviating infertility is *in vitro fertilization* (IVF). In this technique a ripe egg is extracted from the ovary, mixed with semen, and then transferred to the uterus of the carrying mother. The technique of *in vitro* fertilization creates many possibilities:

1. Husband's sperm plus wife's egg re-implanted in wife.
2. Donor's sperm plus wife's egg re-implanted in wife.
3. Donor's sperm or husband's sperm plus wife's egg re-implanted in third party (surrogacy).

Clearly, these cases all raise different moral issues, but there are two arguments which are sometimes used against any kind of IVF. The first is that the whole practice is *unnatural*. The trouble with this sort of argument, which is used in many contexts, is that it is difficult to be sure what the terms 'natural' and 'unnatural' mean. Sometimes they refer to what God has ordained, but there seems no unambiguous method of discovering what God's views might be on a specific medical technique. At other times the 'natural' is thought to be what occurs without human interference. But on this reckoning the whole practice of medicine is unnatural. A third view, going back to the Greeks, sees the natural as what leads to the fulfilling of the ends or capacities of human nature. On this interpretation there is a case for saying that techniques which may alleviate infertility do fulfil some of the ends of human nature. Our own view is that the terms 'natural' or 'unnatural' are really terms of rhetoric rather than argument and that they do not help to make out a case one way or the other. (See p. 127.)

A much stronger argument concerns the funding of research into IVF. It can be argued that there are better uses of the money in the life-saving medical services. We deal with general economic arguments in Chapter 17, but note at this point that there are strong scientific and economic considerations in favour of the development of IVF.

- What importance do you attach to the funding of research into techniques for alleviating infertility, as opposed to geriatrics, cancer, multiple sclerosis?

- What are the ethical reasons for and against treatment for infertility being available on the NHS? Is it an illness?

3. SURPLUS EMBRYOS

As so far described the moral problems attached to the use of IVF techniques are not so very different from those associated with AIH or AID. In other words, if IVF simply involves the fertilization *in vitro* by a husband's sperm of an egg extracted from and re-implanted into his wife's uterus then we have simply a morally acceptable extension of infertility services. If the sperm is from a donor the additional problems are those connected with the possible effects on the child. (Surrogacy we shall discuss later.) Unfortunately, the technical and moral problems are more complicated than that. The technical problems arise over difficulties connected with re-implantation. To minimize these difficulties it is common practice to transfer several embryos to the potential mother, thus increasing the chances of pregnancy. There are two moral problems arising from this.

The first is that a multiple pregnancy may result, with the risks of miscarriage or immaturity at birth, and social stress resulting from the live birth of several babies. Such risks must clearly be fully explained to anyone seeking IVF. The second problem is much more controversial from the moral point of view. It concerns the fate of surplus embryos. The surplus embryos are usually frozen and can be used for subsequent pregnancies, but even then there may still be surplus embryos. There seem in that case to be two possibilities — dispose of them, or use them for research or tissue culture. It is precisely these consequences which for many people constitute the crucial moral objection to the use of IVF. The argument can be set out as follows:

If IVF continues then (for the foreseeable future) supplies of embryos surplus to requirements will exist. But it is always wrong to research on or dispose of human embryos. Therefore IVF must be rejected as morally wrong since it necessarily gives rise to what is wrong.

4. CONSENSUS ARGUMENTS ON IVF

Before embarking on a discussion of the moral issues raised by the fate of surplus embryos we should be clear what problem we are addressing in this section. The problems we discussed in Chapter 5, section 1, were philosophical ones and concerned fundamental questions such as:

When does life begin?
When does life have a moral significance?
Does an embryo have moral rights?

Now the Warnock Committee, while it clearly bore these and similar questions in mind, was mainly concerned with a different matter — making recommendations to the Government for legislation. Our community has diverse values and there is unlikely to be unanimity on philosophical and theological questions, but it was the hope of the Warnock Committee that there could be a *consensus* view. A consensus view may be obtained (when it can) by consulting a wide range of opinion (as the Warnock Committee did) and trying to sift it for common elements. Another method of creating consensus is by drawing attention to other practices or techniques which are widely accepted but which do not differ in principle from what is in dispute. In this case these other practices are abortion and contraceptive techniques using the 'morning-after' pill or intra-uterine devices (IUD) which allow fertilization but prevent implantation. The argument now becomes:

> If IVF is to be considered morally wrong, then the use of IUD and abortion must be considered wrong for the same reason (they all lead to the death of the embryo). But there is a consensus accepting the latter practices, so there must in consistency be an acceptance of the former.

If this consensus approach is accepted then the health care professions are left with the different (and non-moral) problem of presenting the issues to the public so that they can become used to them and not see them in the wrong light. It is important to note about the consensus argument (and the Warnock Committee Report) that it, in effect and perhaps rightly, side-steps the question of whether these practices *are* wrong. The same is true of any consensus argument.

Now even if we suppose that there is a consensus for IUD contraceptive methods and abortion, that would establish at most only that we cannot in logic condemn the *disposal* of surplus embryos; there might still be a consensus to condemn *experimenting* on them. In fact, there are two special arguments against experimenting on embryos which do not apply to disposing of them.

The first of these arguments draws an analogy with war. It is considered permissible to kill in war, but not to experiment on prisoners of war. But this is a poor analogy. Adults can feel pain and fear but embryos at this early stage cannot (see pp. 65–7).

The second argument is a stronger one. It is the 'slippery slope' argument (see pp. 129–30). In general terms the argument is that while doing 'a' may be permissible it will lead to the doing of b, c, d . . . and at some stage we reach a practice which is definitely wrong. Applying this to the possibility of embryo experiments the argument would be that by accepting such experiments we are breaking a taboo and placing ourselves on a slippery slope leading to experiments on the mentally retarded and so on. Therefore we ought not to put a foot on the slope.

Against this we might first note that the argument does not assert that embryo experiments are wrong, but only that by breaking a taboo they may lead to our acceptance of what is wrong. This consequentialist argument could be countered if there were strong consequentialist considerations in favour of embryo research. Let us consider these. They are the economic and scientific considerations referred to at the beginning of our discussion of IVF.

One argument is that we ought to make use of surplus embryos for the good of mankind, for it seems clear that a vast amount of good can come from such experiments. For example, it has been asserted that genetic diseases might be eliminated within a few generations. Again, there are possibilities of growing organs for transplants, and these will bring benefits to medicine.

A second argument, which is weak on its own, can be added to strengthen the first if the first is accepted. It is that the benefits mentioned in the first argument are widely recognized and that experiments on embryos are going to take place whether we approve or not. It is therefore important to *control* these experiments and the experimenters, rather than ban them completely. To this end the Warnock Committee allowed experiments only until 14 days and then only by licensed experimenters.

A third argument is that such experiments will cut down on the need for experiments on animals. This has two benefits, the technical one that it minimizes the reliance on extrapolation from the animal to the human, and the moral one that it cuts down on animal suffering. There is an increasing body of public opinion which attaches weight to this last consideration and it therefore can be added to the consensus in favour of allowing experiments on embryos. (See also Chapter 8, section 1.)

IVF is a much more controversial technique than AIH or AID because it requires the creation of surplus human embryos, which must in the end be disposed of or become objects of experimentation. This is likely to be regarded as wrong unless it is carefully described and seen to be no different in principle from certain contraceptive practices widely accepted. There may also be a consensus for experimentation on embryos when the enormous advantages for human welfare are appreciated.

- What do you think of the use of consensus arguments?
- Do you think there is a significant moral difference between disposing of surplus embryos and using them for research?
- Do you think it is morally better to use human embryos up to 14 days for research or to use mature animals?
- Do you think it right to *create* embryos for the sole purpose of research?

Read again the relevant sections on persons and respect in Chapter 4, section 2, and Chapter 5, section 1.

- Do you think the morally important question is − 'When does life begin?'?
- Will scientists one day discover exactly when an embryo becomes a person?
- What are the arguments for and against the view that the embryo is potentially a person, so should be accorded the rights of a person?

5. ABORTION

It should be noted here that any view on the status of the embryo has important implications for an abortion policy. It will follow from this position that abortion becomes harder to defend from the moral point of view around eight weeks, for it is around then that the brain develops. This does not mean that abortion would always be wrong when the brain has begun to develop in the embryo; it means only that the wishes of the mother could never be the only consideration. There may sometimes be factors concerning the mother's health or social situation which could be weighed against the rights of the embryo whose brain was developed. But an argument of this kind is not simply about the importance of live tissue within the uterus: it is a matter of weighing the rights of the mother against the rights of the embryo. There are, of course, many other arguments concerned with the rights and wrongs of abortion, but we do not propose to go into these, since they are perhaps the best known of all arguments in the field of health care. But we have included some questions for discussion on the more general aspects of abortion.

- Do you think that there is a moral difference between abortion before 8 weeks and abortion at 12 weeks?
- Suppose that pre-natal diagnosis showed that the embryo had certain defects. List the defects that you would consider good grounds for an abortion.
- Do you consider social circumstances give good grounds for abortion? If so, what circumstances?
- Suppose pre-natal examination disclosed that the baby would be a girl and the mother already had four girls and wanted a boy. Would this constitute good grounds for abortion?
- Do you think that sex determination should be a widely available service?

6. SURROGACY

Less well known are the arguments for and against surrogacy. In this context a surrogate mother is one who has brought to term the fertilized egg of another couple and who then hands over the baby to the other couple to nurture. The Warnock Committee came down against surrogacy on the grounds that it was always liable to commercial exploitation. They recommended that it should be made a criminal offence to create agencies whose purpose is to recruit women for surrogate pregnancy and that even private surrogacy arrangements should not be enforceable by the courts.

Even if this conclusion is not disputed the grounds given by the Warnock Committee for the conclusion seem weak. They argue: 'that people should treat others as a means to their own ends, however desirable the consequences, must always be liable to moral objection. Such treatment of one person by another becomes positively exploitive when financial interests are involved' (8.17). No doubt the members of the Committee went to its meetings by train, aeroplane, or taxi, thereby treating others as a means and involving the exchange of money! The Kantian doctrine is that a person should never be treated *only* as a means but always at the same time as an end; and there seems no clear reason on the face of it why a surrogate mother should not be treated both as a means to aid the infertility of another woman and also as an end − *especially* if she is well paid for it!

The strongest argument against surrogacy refers to the problems of identity which are likely to be created for the child issuing from such an arrangement. Relevant to this is a brief discussion in the Report of perplexing questions of who the 'true' mother is. The Committee saw the options as that the 'true' mother is either the genetic mother or the carrying mother and rules (6.8) 'that when a child is born to a woman following donation of another's egg the woman giving birth should, for all purposes, be regarded in law as the mother of that child, and that the egg donor should have no rights or obligations in respect of the child'.

It would follow from this that the surrogate mother would be the 'true' mother and surrogacy can then be represented as an arrangement in which the 'true' mother is giving away her child for money. No wonder the Committee came down against surrogacy!

Another point of view on origins is sometimes stressed by social workers in adoption agencies − the importance for children of knowing their genetic parents. We must also remember the importance of the *nurturing* mother, who could be different from either the genetic or the carrying mother. Such complications which easily arise over surrogacy cannot be good for the psychology of anyone.

It is therefore possible to accept the conclusion of the Warnock Committee that commercial agencies for surrogacy should be prohibited by law, on the basis of the psychological problems facing a child of such an arrangement rather than on the possibility of exploitation.

● Are there situations in which *you* think surrogacy might be morally permissible (e.g. one sister helping another)?

- If you answer 'Yes' to the preceding question, does it make any moral difference if the surrogate mother is given expenses and some fee for her time and inconvenience?
- If your answer is 'No', do you think there is any difference between offering or hiring your body for surrogacy and giving or selling an organ, your body, or your blood?
- Is there an important moral difference between surrogacy and 'wet nursing'?

7. CONTRACEPTION

The possibility of contraception has been with us for much longer than that of surrogacy, and we do not intend here to rehearse the arguments for and against the practice in general. Recently, however, new forms of contraception coupled with early sexual maturity have given rise to moral problems. One of these concerns the dilemma facing a GP when an under-age girl requests a prescription for a contraceptive pill, especially if she also requests that her parents are not told. This is a medical problem only to the extent that some sorts of pill might not be good for some girls with certain health conditions, but the main problem facing the doctor is a moral one. The doctor will be aware that if he refuses to grant the prescription the 'patient' may either proceed without contraception or go to another doctor. There have been attempts to solve this moral problem by legal means. By taking the issue to the courts it is assumed that legislation will make it lawful or unlawful to prescribe the contraceptive pill to girl。 who are under age. Thus, the general question of the law being used to deal with moral problems is raised.

A connected problem is that of the sexual activity of the mentally handicapped or the slightly subnormal. The special difficulty here is that the person may not understand the instructions or remember to take the pill. For this reason it is tempting to consider prescribing injections such as Depo-Provera which last for a period of months. There are, however, health risks attached to such injections.

Attempting to answer some of the problems in the examples will perhaps enable the reader to come to terms with his/her own views.

- If *you* think that something is morally wrong (abortion, contraception) would you be willing to use it for a patient who does *not* think it wrong?
- If you think that something is morally wrong and are unwilling to prescribe it would you recommend another doctor who would be willing?
- Do you think that sexual activity should be permitted between patients in psychiatric hospitals?
- Would you recommend or persuade someone who was mentally subnormal and sexually active to be sterilized?
- If a woman of 25 with two children wished to be sterilized would you agree?
- If she had no children but was 30 and had a successful career (e.g. in nursing or medicine) would you agree?
- If a childless couple of 30 who had voluntarily terminated their fertility (e.g. with vasectomy or sterilization) subsequently wished to adopt a child, would you regard them as good candidates?
- Issues of abortion, contraception, *in vitro* fertilization, raise the question whether the law should be used to solve ethical and moral problems. Do you think committees, councils, or courts should be used for this purpose?

8. CONCLUSION

Artificial reproduction is an especially good example of an area in which technological advance has taken us by surprise. But admiration for scientific advances easily gives way to anxiety that the human intellect is outstripping human moral sensibilities. It is important that moral discussion, especially by health care professionals, should enable us to relate reproductive technology to our deepest moral sentiments and enable society to decide what can be assimilated into our moral traditions and what rejected.

Chapter 14

QUALITY OF LIFE

As an idea or a concept, the term 'quality of life' is widespread, yet it is difficult to define and interpret for there are many different ways of thinking about it. This was recognized by Aristotle in his *Nicomachean Ethics* when he said,

> . . . when it comes to saying in what happiness consists, opinions differ, and the account given by the generality of mankind is not at all like that of the wise. The former take it to be something obvious and familiar, like pleasure or money or eminence and there are various other views, and often the same person actually changes his opinion. When he falls ill he says that it is health, and when he is hard up he says that it is money.*

1. DEFINITIONS AND DIMENSIONS OF QUALITY OF LIFE

Over the years, many attempts have been made to define quality of life. The fact that none is universally acceptable indicates the difficulty of the task. Most, however, would agree that quality if life relates to the individual person, that it is best perceived by that person, that conceptions of it change with time, and that it must be related to all aspects of life. Thus, a 'good' quality of

*Book 1, Chapter 4.

life may mean different things to different people, and, with the passage of time, the things that matter may change. This is particularly the case when illness occurs. One way of looking at quality of life is to consider the differences between the hopes and ambitions of the individual, and the actual state he or she is in. In terms of this definition the process of achieving a good quality of life means narrowing the gap between hopes and reality. This implies that individual personal growth must occur to achieve a good quality of life.

As we have maintained, quality of life is concerned not just with the presence or absence of physical illness but with many other dimensions. These include work and leisure, interpersonal relationships between family and friends, psychological and emotional aspects of life, including coping with illness and treatment, and spiritual aspects of life. These are just a few of the dimensions which can be considered to be important in 'quality of life'.

- List for yourself those areas which you consider to be important for *your* own life.
- Do you think you could *measure* your quality of life?

Definitions and dimensions, however adequate, do not help if they do not give guidance to the patient or the health care team. As has been discussed in other sections, information and knowledge of treatment and procedures are necessary to assist in making health care decisions. The knowledge-base is important, but attitudes and values are also critical.

Suppose for example that in the treatment of a particular condition, two procedures are available.

1. Procedure A involves a six-month course of injections and medication, during which time the patient will experience considerable side-effects which will definitely affect the 'quality of life'. It does, however, give the patient a 70 per cent chance of surviving five years.
2. Procedure B involves a course of medication which has minimal side-effects, but the chance of survival at five years is less than 10 per cent.

- The question here is to define those factors *in this patient* which would make you decide, in association with the patient, which treatment to use.

Take two patients, both suffering from arthritis, and of the same severity:

Patient 1. A 35-year-old woman with two children.
Patient 2. A 70-year-old woman living on her own.

Try to answer the following questions.

- Which factors would be important in determining the treatment used? What further information might you require?
- Would you consider that the age and social status of the patient should be taken into account?
- How much would you involve the patient and the family in the decision?
- How would you try to measure quality of life in these two patients?
- How much would the quality of life of the family, as opposed to the patient, be taken into account?

Look at another example. An elderly man has recently had a stroke. He has been rehabilitated but cannot feed himself and requires assistance for toilet functions. There are no economic reasons, or pressure on beds, to prevent his staying in hospital, but both he and his wife wish to be at home together. The team agrees with this decision in principle but it is clear that the wife is not in good health and, in addition, it will only be possible to provide a community nursing service for two hours a day, meals on wheels, and a home help.

- What additional information would you need to make a decision about sending him home?
- How much should *her* quality of life be taken into account?
- List the arguments for and against keeping him in hospital.
- If you decide to send him home, how will you monitor his 'quality of life'? List five aspects you would check.

Physical and mental handicap in children is another area in which 'quality of life' is frequently discussed. Take Alison, a child born with severe spina bifida. She is paralysed from the waist down and has no control over bowel or bladder function. At the age of one year she has already had a series of life-threatening infections and has been hospitalized for 50 per cent of the year. The parents are devoted to their daughter, and have two other children aged three and five years. Alison has just been admitted with a severe urinary tract infection.

- How would you assess the quality of life of the patient, the parents, and the other children?
- List the arguments for and against active treatment of this infective episode.
- What right have (i) the health care team, (ii) the parents, to make decisions about treatment based on the quality of life?

2. HYPOTHESES

In Chapter 11, section 2, there was a discussion on the management of uncertainty, and we have discussed hypotheses in science in Chapter 2, section 2. With quality of life, many of the decisions we make relate to this uncertainty. In some instances the decisions may be immediate, urgent and of a 'life and death' nature. Many, however, will not be so urgent and there will be time for reflection and thought. In these cases there is the possibility of using hypotheses or, in other words, of *trying* a particular course of action and evaluating the outcome. This is the basis of many aspects of medical and nursing practice. The situation is assessed, the management planned and implemented and the course of action evaluated. In other words:

1. A hypothesis is set up and tested.
2. It is possible to *change* the course of action if it does not succeed.

Look again at the case of the elderly man with the stroke who wishes to go home. Instead of making a decision, yes or no, the hypothesis could be tested. Let's send him home and see. If things work out well, then he can stay, but if it proves difficult for his wife then he may require hospitalization again.

The key feature here is that instead of making absolute value judgements in situations of uncertainty which might be considered irreversible, tentative judgements can be made which can then be reviewed and revised. This is of particular relevance when the members of the team disagree as to the plan of action. Since such decisions are usually based on judgements or assessments with incomplete facts, then it is possible *openly* to try one course of action recognizing that this may be changed. In this way the whole team can use this problem as a learning situation.

3. QUANTITY AND QUALITY

A distinction is often drawn between the quantity of life (for example the length of survival) and the quality of life. There is often the implication that people in whom the quantity of life is improved by treatment may suffer a decrease in quality of life. This is a notion which must be questioned. If survival is improved (for example if the patient is cured) then the quality of life is also likely to be improved.

Two phrases are often used in this connection: 'adding years to life', and 'adding life to years'. This is sometimes described as the 'compression of morbidity', which means that the objective of increasing life-span should be associated at the same time with an increasing quality of life or reduction of disability.

Where there are conflicts, it is in relation to treatments which do *not* improve quantity (i.e. which are ineffective) and may well reduce quality of life. Since uncertainty as to the outcome is almost always present it does require judgement as to the most likely outcome. We noted in the previous section that it is possible to test this hypothesis, with the full consent of the patient, and to reverse the decisions if the treatment proves ineffective or if side-effects are severe. In this case the patient has a *chance* that long-term benefit will result. In this discussion it has been assumed, of course, that the treatment is reversible, and this clearly does not apply to some surgical procedures.

A discussion of the quantity and quality of life inevitably raises the *economic* aspects of health care. If resources are scarce then procedures which might improve the quality of life of a patient may be denied for financial reasons. In the assessment of the value of procedures, quality of life is increasingly taken into account. We shall go into the economic aspects of health care in more detail in Chapter 17.

4. THE CONTROL OF ILLNESS

In the overall control of illness and the maintenance of health, prevention and early diagnosis are the keys to success, but in those patients who do become ill, and who therefore may require treatment, there are three possible objectives which are often confused yet have a direct bearing on the quality of life. These objectives are:

1. To cure the illness and eliminate the disease. In minor illnesses, this is not particularly difficult. The chronic diseases (cancer, heart disease, stroke), however, may present much more of a problem. For many patients, therefore, cure may not be the objective of treatment.

2. To control the illness by reducing the symptoms or by restoring normality for a period of time: months, years, or decades. In the chronic illnesses this may be the major objective.

3. To improve the quality of life. Naturally, in relation to 1 and 2 above, if the treatment used is 'successful' then it is likely that the quality of life will also be improved. To improve quality of life alone, without affecting quantity, is a legitimate objective on its own.

Problems in individual patients tend to occur if these objectives are confused and not thought through. They are not mutually exclusive and there may be movement between objectives.

- Give some examples of diseases or illness or situations where you think:
    - (a) the disease is curable;
    - (b) the illness requires control;
    - (c) illnesses or situations in which the overriding concern is for quality of life.

- When you have made this list can you determine for yourself the reasons why you listed them in the different categories?

5. QUALITY OF LIFE OF STAFF

This is an issue which is not often discussed, but is one of considerable importance. Dealing on a day-to-day basis with ill people can not only have an important effect on the health care professional which can affect his or her clinical decision-making capacity, but also can affect family and friends. Health can also suffer and it is therefore very important that steps are taken not to compromise the quality of life of the carer. (Read Chapter 4, section 3; Chapter 12, section 10.)

6. CONCLUSION

Quality of life is an idea which it is difficult to do without in health care, and yet it is a source of embarrassment because it is also difficult to make precise and to quantify. It is related on the one hand to objective features of health and welfare − such as freedom from pain or discomfort, mobility, abilities to think, read, talk, etc. − and on the other hand to more subjective reactions such as the individual's toleration of the absence of such features and his hopes of recovering them. It is this combination of the objective and the subjective which makes the idea both hard to analyse and impossible to discard.

Chapter 15
PUBLIC HEALTH:
THE MORAL ISSUES

1. INDIVIDUAL AND COMMUNITY

So far in this part of the book, we have been concerned with the
individual, his or her rights, quality of life, etc. In health care,
however, there is another dimension, that of the community.
Important factors in this discussion include the resources
available in the community and the differences between different
geographical areas. They also include the important topics of
information given to the public, the question of prevention, early
diagnosis and screening. Some aspects related to the community
will also be discussed in the chapter on economic issues. (Read
also Chapter 6, sections 4, 5, 6.)

It should be clear that in some instances the health of the community may conflict with that of the individual. For example,
if we take patients with infectious disease it is possible to
make the case that such individuals should be isolated to protect
the rest of the community. This may impinge on individual
rights and could mean loss of employment and separation from
the family. It may even mean treatment, even though the infected individual may apparently have no sign of the illness. For
example, a patient who is a carrier of salmonella, an organism
responsible for food poisoning, may be asymptomatic yet cause

considerable harm. Infective hepatitis as a source of potential harm to health care workers is well known. In more recent times the increase in the incidence of AIDS and HIV infection has raised even broader issues about the individual's health and that of the wider community. The possibility of infection of, for instance, dentists by patients with AIDS or hepatitis B is a real one, and there is a serious moral problem as to whether potentially infective patients should be identified and those caring for them informed. This could be regarded as putting the label 'unclean' on such individuals, but what of the risk to others? With this in mind the following questions might be asked.

- How do you justify infringing the liberty of the individual to improve the health of others?
- In what circumstances would you consider it necessary to isolate individuals from the community?
- What restrictions, if any, would you place on individuals who are potentially a danger to the health of the community?

2. VACCINATION

Vaccination against specific diseases potentially confers great benefit on the community. On the other hand there is often a risk to the individual. It may be necessary therefore to ask for consent before vaccination is carried out. Read the section on consent (Chapter 18, section 3) and ask yourself:

- Is consent required before vaccination?
- Would your views change in the case of a common disease in a tropical country?
- If consent is required, how much information would you give on the potential harmful effects? Would you include the mortality risks?

The topics of prevention and screening will be discussed in subsequent parts of this chapter.

3. ADVERTISING AND THE COMMUNITY

In a wider sense the messages which the public obtain from the media may be relevant to the health of the community. The most obvious example is cigarette smoking, where the evidence for a health hazard is overwhelming.

Alcohol advertising is a further example. In a world-wide sense there is the introduction of such habits into Third World countries which could be considered to be morally wrong. It is necessary to analyse carefully each of these situations before making moral judgements. Here are some questions you might ask yourself:

- What are the arguments for and against cigarette advertising? Should it be allowed at sporting events?
- Should advertising of alcoholic products be banned? If not, why not?
- What steps would you take to influence the advertising of cigarettes in a Third World country?

4. HEALTH AND POLITICAL ISSUES

We have emphasized in this book the intimate relationship between the health worker as a professional and as an individual public citizen. Nothing highlights this better than health-related political issues where the doctor or nurse may be involved as an individual as well as a professional.

- Take the issue of nuclear waste. How far should the professional be involved in such issues? As a doctor − or as an individual? Is it possible to separate the two?
- Suppose that your children attend the local primary school, and there is some evidence that asbestos tiles have been used in the roofing. You, as a parent, but also as a professional, are asked to be part of the committee to take action on the matter. In what circumstances would you agree to take part? What would your role be − a professional, a parent, a public citizen?

5. SMOKING AND HEALTH

This topic provides a fascinating problem in relation to the health of the individual versus that of the community at large. There is very good evidence now that cigarette smoking has major adverse effects on health. Doctors and other professionals have a duty to point this out to patients and the public. However, there is a difficult question as to how hard the doctor should try to stop the patient from smoking without infringing individual freedom.

● Consider the following courses of action and decide which of them would be reasonable, faced with a patient who smokes cigarettes.
  1. Take no action at all.
  2. Give general advice on the dangers of smoking.
  3. Suggest attendance at an anti-smoking group.
  4. Emphasize the impact on relatives of premature death related to smoking.
  5. Say that you will not see the patient again unless smoking stops.

There is also evidence that cigarette smoking can be harmful to non-smokers who are exposed to cigarette smoke. The evidence comes from the incidence of illness in the children and spouses of smokers. Thus, while individuals have a right to smoke if they wish, there is a conflict if they interfere with the health of others. For example, in a hospital waiting room or dayroom area smoking is often permitted, yet non-smokers may suffer as a result.

● How would you argue for and against cigarette smoking in communal hospital areas or other public spaces? Consider the rights of the individual versus the public at large.

Another argument can also be introduced at this stage, that of the economic effects of cigarette smoking. On the one hand there is a case for saying that the income from the taxing of cigarette purchase is very important in keeping the health service functioning. On the other there is the cost to the health service of treating those patients who develop smoking related diseases. Further, there is the time lost from work because of illness which affects productivity.

- Consider the arguments for and against reducing the income to the country by a successful campaign to stop smoking versus the reduction in the costs of treatment. Bear in mind the time-scale of this. There is an argument for increasing the tax on tobacco by a substantial amount. Is this fair to those who smoke and have a right to do so if they wish?

6. PREVENTION

Prevention is the key to the control of many illnesses and it is likely to become more important in the future. All health care professionals should have a role in prevention. In the prevention of illness several approaches may be used.

The *first* is an alteration of life-style, which would involve such factors as cigarette smoking, diet, and exercise. A *second* approach is to identify groups at high risk of developing a particular illness and to follow them closely and if necessary intervene. For example, there are a number of conditions such as ulcerative colitis and colonic polyps which are known to predispose to large bowel cancer. Having identified high-risk patients, doctors can monitor their progress. But several interesting moral questions arise including:

- Should patients be informed that they are at high risk of developing a particular illness or disease?
- Suppose that we know that there is a risk of a benign bowel polyp changing and becoming malignant, but the patient refuses an operation to remove it. What would you say?

A *third* approach is to use some form of vaccination procedure. This has been extremely successful in eliminating a range of previously very serious or fatal diseases. There is a price however — that of the potential side-effects of the vaccination itself. Such side-effects are well recorded and can result in death or severe handicap. There comes a time, therefore, where decisions about the use of vaccine must be made.

- Suppose that a vaccine for a common illness is available. The disease itself is minor in most patients but in some the disease can cause severe respiratory problems and there is an associated mortality. For the disease the morbidity is 1 in 10 000, the mortality is 1 in 50 000. The vaccine is also associated with morbidity and mortality. At what level do you think the use of the vaccine would be acceptable?

1 in 5000 morbidity	1 in 10 000 mortality
1 in 10 000 morbidity	1 in 50 000 mortality
1 in 20 000 morbidity	1 in 70 000 mortality
1 in 50 000 morbidity	1 in 100 000 mortality

7. SCREENING

Screening for disease seems to make sense. It makes possible the identification of the illness at an early stage, when treatment can be started with the hope of long-term cure. Predisposing factors can be identified and, if possible, eliminated. There are, however, several problems associated with screening programmes.

1. *The false negative test.* In this instance the test has been normal, but it has failed to pick up the disease. The patient may have been given the 'all-clear'.

2. *The false positive test.* The test suggests that a particular disease is present, but subsequent investigation does not confirm this.

3. *Ineffective treatment for the disease.* This is a particular problem. The test is abnormal, but the treatment is ineffective.

4. *High risk groups who do not come for screening.* There is some evidence in cervical cancer that those at high risk belong

to those with a low socio-economic status, and such groups are the very ones who do not use screening services.

Particular examples of the problems associated with screening are exemplified by the following case-history. As part of a routine screening survey a series of blood tests are performed on otherwise normal healthy individuals. One of these tests measures the serum level of gamma glutamyl transferase (GT), which may be elevated in conditions of abnormal liver function, notably related to alcoholic liver damage, but may in some cases be normal. Conversely, as in all blood tests, there is a 'normal' range and some 'normal' patients have levels which fall out of this range.

• A 52-year-old, otherwise fit man who has been admitted for repair of an inguinal hernia, has a blood test which reports an elevated level of GT. The patient is *not* told about this but is asked to return and a second blood sample is taken, which confirms the elevated level. To investigate this fully would require a number of other tests, including a liver biopsy. Because the test is abnormal he is referred to you.

1. What would you tell the patient?
2. Would you investigate the patient further or would you wait a few months and repeat the test?
3. Would you raise the question of a history of excessive alcohol intake?

A similar sequence of events might occur in the diagnosis and management of hypertension. There is still controversy as to what level of elevated blood pressure requires treatment.

• Suppose that you are a general practitioner who, on routine examination of a 35-year-old woman, detects an elevated blood pressure 140/100. She is otherwise asymptomatic. A repeat visit is arranged and the level is 140/95, still elevated a little. Would you tell the patient?

• It is possible in this age-group that there is a remediable cause, but this would require hospital admission and investigation, which might carry a morbidity or even a mortality. If you were the patient, and were given this information, would you wish further investigations to be done or would your choice be to live with the slightly elevated blood pressure?

8. PREDICTING HEALTH

As our understanding of the genetic basis of health and disease grows it will become possible to predict, in some instances, patterns of disease or illness. Already it is possible in the unborn child, using a series of tests, to predict sex, and in some cases outcome screening is already available for a number of diseases by testing *in utero*. This is likely to be increasingly available. While no intrinsically new moral problems are raised, a number of important topics need to be considered:

● When testing the genetic profile of an individual, whose property is the result, and how may the information be disseminated?

● As testing of the unborn child for genetic influences progresses, would you put limits on the process?

9. INEQUALITIES IN HEALTH CARE

It does not take a great deal of careful observation to note that some areas of the country are better served by health services than others. This may relate to specialist services or to community care. For example, one district may have a specialist renal dialysis service, but no hospice for the continuing care of the terminally ill. Another may have a community based diabetic service, but no cardiac surgery. Such inequalities have often grown up by chance, related to the interest of a particular professional group. These inequalities, however, do raise important moral issues as well as economic ones.

- Do all members of the community have the right to have access to specialist services provided within the local area?
- Should some services be centralized and not available locally?
- What is the minimum which should be provided locally? — maternity care, child care, renal transplantation, radio-therapy, etc.?

This issue will be discussed further in Chapter 17.

10. CONCLUSION

From this brief review it can be seen that community aspects of health raise a number of important moral issues. In some cases it is not possible to separate the role of the professional from that of his role as a public citizen. Screening raises very general issues about truth-telling which were discussed in Chapter 10.

Chapter 16

A QUESTION OF DYING

Death and dying are emotive issues and among the subjects most commonly discussed when moral questions are raised. They involve such major issues as euthanasia, suicide, resuscitation, and terminal care, and include both sudden death and death from chronic illness. The questions of truth-telling, quality of life, consent, teamwork, and many others need to be considered, and some of these are discussed elsewhere in this book. Just as there are moral problems in defining when life begins, so are there problems in defining when life ends. These are important in the consideration of brain death and the use of organs for transplantation.

This chapter, therefore, will deal with a series of topics relation to the question of death and dying. It is important, however, that they are not seen in isolation; rather they are related to the other topics and concepts raised in this book.

1. THE DEFINITION OF DEATH

In conventional terms, and for the vast majority of patients, death is said to occur when respiration ceases, followed by cessation of the heart beat. These changes are diagnosed by simple clinical methods. Such observations were sufficient until developments in medical care made it necessary to look more closely at this method of determining death. These developments included:

1. The ability to maintain adequate respiration indefinitely by artificial means.

2. The need for donor organs in a satisfactory condition for the purposes of transplantation.

These developments gave rise to the moral problem as to whether respiration should be maintained artificially when there was evidence of damage to other organs, notably the brain. It was for this reason that agreed criteria for making the diagnosis of brain death have gradually evolved over the last 20 years. The objective of these criteria is to establish that the patient has irreversible brain damage, due to injury or haemorrhage.

There are slight variations in the criteria which are used in different countries but most include:

1. Exclusion of other causes of brain damage which might be reversible.
2. Absence of brainstem reflexes. The corneal, pupillary contraction, and oculo-vestibular reflexes are tested.
3. No spontaneous respiration. To test for this the ventilator is switched off for five minutes and the patient observed. During this time oxygenation is maintained.
4. Laboratory tests, notably electroencephalography (EEG) which records electrical current in the brain. As both false positive and false negative recordings can occur, most doctors recognize that the EEG is not required for making the diagnosis.

When the diagnosis of brain death is confirmed in the manner described above, the ventilator may then be switched off.

Making the diagnosis of brain death and the switching off of the ventilator raises many moral questions. Let us assume that an 18-year-old has sustained a head injury in a motor cycle accident. After his admission to a neurosurgical unit and stabilization of his condition, the tests described above are carried out and the diagnosis of brain death is made. The family has been informed of the patient's condition.

● Do you think that doctors, nurses or other professionals have any right to switch off the ventilator?

- What would be the consequences, good or bad, of keeping the respiratory support going?
- Are you personally satisfied with the criteria given above?

It has been decided that, following the diagnosis of brain death, the patient's kidneys will be used for the purposes of transplantation.

- What are the moral arguments for, and against, the use of cadaveric organs for transplantation?
- What form of consent do you think is necessary.
- Do you make any *moral* distinctions between the use of skin, cornea, kidney, liver, or heart, for the purposes of transplantation?
- What are the moral differences between the use of live donors and cadaveric donors in transplantation?

Contracting in and contracting out: As donors are urgently required for the purposes of transplantation, members of the public are asked to carry with them donor cards. Such cards express a positive wish on behalf of the individual to donate his or her organs in the event of death occurring. Several moral issues are raised by carrying such cards.

- For example, suppose that an individual is carrying a kidney donor card, and dies suddenly as the result of an accident. The relatives are informed but *they* refuse to allow the organs to be used. Whose wishes should be respected?

Another possible approach to the issue is that members of the public should take one of two courses of action.

1. *They could contract in*: A central register would be kept of all who were willing to have their organs used in the event of death. This would also mean that those who had not put their names on the register would not have organs removed.

2. *They could contract out*: A positive decision would be made to say 'no' to organ donation in the event of death. This would also mean that those who had not made this positive

decision to opt out could have their organs removed without permission.

- What do you think of these schemes?

2. THE QUESTION OF RESUSCITATION

In the course of clinical practice in hospital and the community, sudden deaths occur. Many of these will be related to myocardial infarctions and there is always the possibility of being able to resuscitate such patients by artificial respiration, external cardiac massage, drug therapy, electrical stimulation of the heart and other techniques. Because brain damage can occur within a few minutes of the cardiac arrest it is essential that a decision to resuscitate is taken immediately. As this often falls to the most junior member of staff, nurse, or doctor, who is available at the time before the 'cardiac arrest' team arrives, it has been suggested that guide-lines as to who should be resuscitated should be available, and that this might then be decided before the event occurs. Naturally, a sudden event like this might not be predictable for the individual patient, but for a group of patients in hospital it is *possible* to make such decisions before the event takes place. This of course raises a whole range of moral questions about the subject of resuscitation. Read Chapter 5, section 2, and then answer these questions.

- What factors do you think are important in a decision to resuscitate a patient? Age, sex, disease . . . etc.
- Should general guide-lines be drawn up by individual clinical units as to which classes of patient should, or should not, be resuscitated, or is this a decision to be made about individual patients?
- How should this be communicated within the ward team? Should a note be made in the case-sheet or the nursing charts?
- If so, who should be part of that decision — doctors, nurses, the family, the patient?
- If a patient asks not to be resuscitated what would you say?

The 'living will': For some people concern about resuscitation and the use of extraordinary measures to keep them alive is sufficient for them to draw up a document, sometimes known as the 'living will', which gives their views on such issues and is to be used to advise the team on their wishes. Some people do not want to be resuscitated.

The prolongation of life: It is now possible, because of improvements in technology, to keep individuals alive for long periods of time. This possibility exists even for patients who are in a vegetative state and brain-dead. In addition, in patients who suddenly become unwell as a result of disease or accident, techniques are available which will restore vital functions and keep the patients alive.

- Do you think life should be preserved at all costs?
- If not, why not?
- Is there a distinction between withholding food and withholding treatment?

3. EUTHANASIA

The term euthanasia, which means death without suffering, or a good death, is associated with major moral problems for the health care team. It is not unusual for a doctor during his career to be asked to 'end this suffering' or 'just give me a big blue pill'. It is therefore a very real practical problem, as well as one associated with important philosophical overtones. It is possible to qualify the word euthanasia in four ways, and it is useful to distinguish these at this point.

1. *Voluntary euthanasia*: In this case the patient makes a conscious decision that his or her life should end, and asks for help in doing so. This is sometimes called assisted suicide.

2. *Involuntary euthanasia*: In this instance society, or an individual in society, makes a positive decision to end the life of someone suffering without asking consent from the sufferer.

3. *Active euthanasia*: This implies that some active step, for example the giving of a drug, has been taken to cause the death of the sufferer.

4. *Passive euthanasia*: In this case no *active* treatment is given, rather treatment is withheld. For example, if an infection occurs, this is not treated.

Euthanasia has been discussed in relation to most illnesses and age-groups though most commonly in relation to diseases associated with severe mental or physical disability or in relation to severe suffering, usually pain. Malformed or abnormal children, or those with a terminal illness, are usually the subjects of this discussion. Clearly, the doctor has a general duty to sustain life and to avoid giving patients anything which might harm them. At the same time, however, this should not result in the prolongation of suffering, something which can happen as a consequence of the inappropriate use of mechanical and drug aids to relieve symptoms, such as drips, tubes, and antibiotics. There is the right to live but also the right to die. Here are some questions for discussion in relation to euthanasia.

- Do you think euthanasia should be practised? If your answer is 'yes' or 'no', how would you defend your response?
- Do you make any distinctions between active and passive euthanasia?
- Can you think of circumstances when you would not use antibiotics in certain classes of patient with a known infection which was life-threatening?
- In this respect would you distinguish between the treatment of a physically handicapped child and an elderly man?
- If someone asked you to give her a 'big blue pill' to end all her suffering, how would you respond?
- If a patient says he has a 'right to die' how would you answer?
- If the relatives asked you 'to put an end to his misery', what would you say?

Acts and omissions: In dealing with a dying patient, we have two possibilities to consider. The first is to act to accelerate the process of death. The second is to withhold treatment which could prolong life. This is sometimes put more forcibly as 'killing, or letting die'. It could be thought that it is morally indefensible to 'kill' patients, while withholding treatment is morally acceptable.

- Do you think there is a moral difference between acts and omissions?
- If yes, give your reasons.
- If not, are there no circumstances when you would consider withholding treatment?

The doctrine of double effect: In relation to acts and omissions the doctrine of double effect is often cited. This doctrine asserts that an action can be 'good' if it is intended to achieve a desirable effect, even if it is foreseen that there is a risk of harm resulting. For example, it would be legitimate to increase the dose of an analgesic with the intention of controlling pain, even if the dose used was associated with the foreseen possibility of hastening death. The doctrine states that this action (in spite of the double effect) is still morally justified. Read pp. 130–1 and then consider:

- Do you agree with this doctrine?

4. DEATH WITH DIGNITY

This is a phrase which is frequently used in relation to dealing with dying and terminal illness. It implies that the individual dies, free of tubes, drips, or drugs, conscious and able to take part in events until the end. The picture is one of peace, acceptance, and minimal suffering. It would be fair to say that such events are rarer than we, as professionals, might like. Yet the concept is an important one. It stresses the need for all individuals, living or dying, to be autonomous human beings with rights and feelings, and shows how easily we can strip such things from patients.

Does this mean, however, that all deaths should be like this? What if a patient wished 'to go out fighting' hoping against hope that things might get better? Would you deny this and take the drip down?

- The description given above is a personal one by the authors of what 'death with dignity' means. This is such an important concept that you should have your own view of what it means. Read Chapter 4, section 2, and then define, in your own terms, what 'death with dignity' means.

5. SUICIDE

Suicide is a deliberate act of self-destruction, taking one's own life. For countries in the West there have been strong moral, religious and legal barriers to suicide. Though the law in England and Wales against committing suicide was repealed in the 1960s it is still an offence to aid or abet a person to commit the act. Individuals may be driven to suicide for a variety of reasons including medical ones, such as serious mental or physical illness, or social problems. The moral questions remain. Check Chapter 4, section 2, before answering these questions.

- In what circumstances, if any, would it be right for an individual to take his or her own life?
- Is it necessarily wrong to assist in this?
- While the individual may have solved his problems, friends and relatives remain. What rights do others have in relation to suicide?
- How would you deal with someone who had 'attempted' suicide, but was now well? Would you say that it was morally wrong for him to have tried to take his own life?

6. TERMINAL ILLNESS AND HOSPICES

This term (terminal illness) is normally confined to individuals in whom

(1) the diagnosis has been confirmed;

(2) the death is certain and not too far off;

(3) medical and nursing effort has turned from the curative to the palliative.

This definition emphasizes several important points. The first is that the patient has an illness which is fatal, and not some non-fatal illness which is mimicking the signs and symptoms. For example, it is possible for patients with cancer to develop symptoms such as headache or abdominal pain which may be due to simple conditions as well as spread of the disease. Sometimes sinister symptoms are simple. The second feature is that death is certain and not too far off. We have already emphasized the difficulties of prognosis and dealing with uncertainty. The final point is that terminal illness requires as much activity and intensive care as other periods of illness. This is a stage where patients should not be forgotten, but cared for by the whole team.

Many of the moral issues associated with terminal care have already been raised, or will be discussed elsewhere − for example, truth-telling, consent, the management of uncertainty, quality of life, euthanasia, and several others. These highlight the need for communication skills for all concerned.

One aspect which has not yet been discussed is where special care for such patients should be provided. In general terms, this care is often provided in a hospice.

The hospice movement, as it has often been called, has developed rapidly over the last 20 years or so, and provides care of superb quality for patients who are dying. It has provided the stimulus for research, development, and teaching, and has clearly shown the value of the team approach. Such a movement, however, raises a series of moral questions, which are concerned with many aspects of specialized patient care.

- Should hospices be available in all areas of the country in sufficient numbers to deal with all dying patients?
- Is it right to segregate dying patients from other patients? If your answer is yes or no, try to justify it.

- Does the role which hospices play in present society mean that other staff in the hospital or community do not have the expertise to deal with dying patients?
- Many of the hospices and nursing homes are funded by charitable organizations. Should they be funded by the NHS and, if so, what services would you sacrifice to meet the additional costs?
- Quality of life and quality of care are important concepts. How would you investigate the differences, if any, between hospital care and hospice care of the dying patient?

7. CONCLUSION

Death is an inevitable consequence of life. As such it raises a wide range of moral issues. With the increasing use of technology and the increasingly successful range of treatments available, it is likely that the problems will increase rather than decrease. Many of the attitudes and values of the health professional in relation to death are very personal and relate to their reactions to death itself. In understanding the moral problems surrounding death and dying, perhaps the most important factor is to examine our own feelings about the subject.

Chapter 17

A QUESTION OF ECONOMICS

1. ECONOMICS AND MORALITY

Establishing priorities is an important aspect of everyday life at home or in business. In any situation it is necessary to establish such priorities, but it is especially important in areas of limited resources, such as health care. It follows that it would be of great assistance if it were possible to evaluate the benefits of particular procedures or treatments and to relate these to costs, for this might allow more rational choices to be made. The assumption here is that with a limited amount of resources economic analysis would encourage the most efficient use of these resources for the greatest benefit of the greatest number of people. In other words, economic analysis in health care is required by the principle of utility, which was one of the basic moral principles we discussed in Chapter 4. But economic efficiency may mean using resources for some groups of people and denying them to others, or cutting out some services entirely. Difficult moral choices have therefore to be made and the principle of justice as well as that of utility is relevant.

In clinical practice, economics and morality are closely related. Making decisions about patients or clients almost always commits the use of resources − for example, a return visit from the doctor or the nurse, a prescription, an investigation, an operation, organizing a home help, dietary advice, etc. Indeed, the consultation by the doctor which established the diagnosis, and possible prognosis, and sets out plans for treatment and investigation, is the basic building block of resource allocation and use in the Health Service. Since in any system resources are finite it is necessary that choices have to be made as there will not be enough to satisfy all demands. Resources must therefore be allocated and there will be competition between the various demands. Use of resources (defined here as skills, people, property or public funds) in one area removes them from elsewhere and is what economists call the 'opportunity cost'. Let us examine some of these problems of utility and distributive justice.

2. INEQUALITIES IN HEALTH CARE

It is well recognized that there are differences in the level of care provided locally, nationally, and internationally. Some of these differences have arisen for historical reasons − a hospital or special service has grown up around a particular local need or demand. In other instances special interests of doctors or other health care workers have established a particular skill in a treatment or diagnostic area. Again, these differences may be related to overt or covert political decisions to have a particular form of treatment available in limited places only. This is the case, for example, in open heart surgery where a limited number of centres have been given sufficient resources to carry out the work. This, of course, makes good economic sense − it can be justified in terms of utility − but it does mean that patients outside these areas must travel to the centre for treatment and this raises questions of justice.

Resource allocation may also vary between different sections of health care. For example, the balance of funding between the acute sector of health care (mainly the large hospitals) and the community sector would be one area to consider. Also, there may be inequalities within sectors, and an example of this may be between the resources required for orthopaedic surgery and neonatal paediatrics.

- Can you identify, within your own area of professional interest, examples of inequality of health care?

● What would you wish to do about them? Are your views based on a desire for social justice or for utility?

3. RESOURCE ALLOCATION

One of the basic principles of the Health Service is the assessment of health and health care needs of the population, and from this determining the resources to be allocated to particular parts of the service. This process (in shorthand, the purchasing function) is then used to set up contracts or agreements with hospitals, community units, etc. (providers), who then deliver the service required. This very explicit process means that priorities have to be determined, and the outcomes monitored to ensure that the needs are met. This therefore identifies the importance of outcome measurement in setting problems.

4. SOME BASIC TERMS OF HEALTH ECONOMICS

If we are going to use health economics as an aid to resolving problems of justice and utility in health care we must introduce some basic terms. At the onset it is important to distinguish needs and demands. *Needs* are the actual requirements of the population under review. Such needs may be readily apparent. For example, to control cigarette smoking in the population is a well-recognized need. Needs may also be hidden in that the population as a whole, or sections of that population, do not recognize that the need exists. For example, cervical screening for the detection of early cervical cancer is not perceived as a need by some sections of the community. *Demands* on the other hand are what the community wishes to be provided with. For example, the community may wish to have a range of high technology options available in its local area. Every district general hospital should have a CT scanner, dialysis, and renal transplantation facilities, or the level of geriatric care provided should be such that all who require specialist care can have access to it. It is not difficult to see how competition and conflict can arise in the allocation of resources.

From what had already been discussed, the health care outcome is central in determining priorities, and resource allocation. Measurement of outcomes can be difficult and might be related, for example, to some observable change (e.g. an improvement in an X-ray) which the professional might be pleased with. On the other hand, the patient might not be happy with the same outcome if the treatment was unpleasant. Thus, there is an important issue of outcome for whom. Based on the outcome, the resource consequences can then be determined by economic appraisal, and a decision made by purchasers on resource allocation to providers.

A key phrase in the Health Service is *option appraisal*. This is a technique which aims to review all possible options (including the zero option) before making choices. Economic analysis is part of this process though choices may be based on grounds which are not exclusively financial.

Economic analysis is a way of measuring and displaying costs and benefits, to assist in the making of choice. It has no magic on its own and must use the raw data supplied with all its uncertainties, but it should help to provide a basis for the moral judgements required, though it must be emphasized that such judgements will still be necessary. There are four ways in which an analysis can be made.

1. *Cost analysis*: This measures only the costs, both direct and indirect, associated with a particular procedure. It does not attempt to measure the benefits of the treatment or assess the consequences. It has, therefore, a limited value.

2. *Cost–benefit analysis*: This form of analysis brings together as many of the costs and benefits as possible. These may well include a series of intangibles such as the cost of suffering or the value of improvement in health. The costs and the benefits are measured in financial terms and this is a useful way of comparing two methods of dealing with the same problem.

3. *Cost-effectiveness analysis*: In this instance the costs are measured in financial terms but the benefits, or effectiveness of treatment, are measured in other ways; for example, survival, time off work, relief of symptoms, etc. Thus, it differs from cost—benefit analysis in which the results are expressed in financial terms. As with cost—benefit analysis it can be used to compare the difference between two methods of dealing with the same problem. For example, the method may be used to compare renal dialysis with transplantation in the treatment of end-stage renal disease. But it cannot be used, at least in a simple way, to compare treatment of different problems, such as renal trans-plantation and coronary artery bypass grafting. This is a major drawback with all the techniques mentioned so far: they do not allow priorities to be developed.

4. *Cost—utility analysis*: This is the most commonly used method at the present time, as it allows comparisons to be made between different illnesses and treatments. The assessment is based on the measurement of Quality-Adjusted Life-Years (QALYs) which can compare the relative value of one health state over another. It brings together changes in survival, morbidity and quality of life in a single measure. In this way quite separate procedures or health problems can be looked at and compared. It is equally concerned with quality and quantity and is not just associated with the financial outcome.

Over the last few years a variety of scales, measures, and indices have been developed to assess those factors considered to be the most important. As was said in the discussion of quality of life, such scales include factors like work, recreation, physical and mental suffering, communication, sleep, dependency on others, feeding, bowel and bladder function, and sexual activity. Some of the scales in current use are filled in by staff, others by the patient.

The use of utilities or QALYs allows differences in individual values to be compared on a scale. These utilities may be described (Torrance, 1986):

Cardinal values are assigned to each Health State on a scale that is established by assigning a value of 1.00 to 'being healthy' and 0.0 to 'being dead'. This is referred to as the 'dead–healthy' scale. The utility values reflect the quality of health status and allow morbidity and mortality and improvements to be combined into a single weighted measure, QALYs gained or lost.

There are, of course, several problems in defining these utility values. Judgement is required in the proper identification of the health state for which utilities are required and in the development and validation of appropriate scales.

We hope to have shown even by this brief account of some terms of health economics how economic analysis can provide a valuable way of assessing the outcome of different ways of dealing with health care problems and so dealing with the problems of justice mentioned to begin with. Using QALYs we can combine quality and quantity into a single measure. An economic analysis alone, at this stage in the development of the measures, will not provide all the answers; moral judgement will still be required to evaluate priorities. Again, while economic analysis will help with planning on a population basis (transplantation gives more QALYs than renal dialysis), it may not help on an individual basis where the health care professional is faced by an individual patient.

5. ECONOMIC ISSUES IN CLINICAL PRACTICE

(a) *Measuring outcomes*: Much of the discussion about economics and morality is related to the question of how we measure performance. Measurement could be in relation to operative morality, bed turnover, out-patient clinic attendance, community care, physiotherapy service, etc.

Measuring outcomes depends on knowing what you want to achieve, the objectives; on having the methods of intervention available, treatment, etc.; and on being able to assess results.

Several techniques have been used to measure outcomes.

1. *The nursing process*: A method of defining objectives, planning, assessing and evaluating patient care.

2. *Problem-orientated medical records* (POMR): This method is essentially the same as the nursing process. It involves seeing patients in a 'problem' way, rather than in a 'disease' way. In other words, the aim is to treat the patient as an individual with problems rather than just as a disease process. The records therefore note the patient's *overall* problems and monitor success in treating them.

3. *Medical (clinical) audit*: This involves combinations of the above, and looks at clinical work in a systematic and critical way.

Whatever the process or technique is called there is a much greater need for accountability in the Health Service: a need for doctors, nurses, and other professionals to take part in the process of audit and to establish priorities within the Health Service.

(b) *Wasting resources*: One method by which we can help to save money is to look at the way we waste resources, either in the hospital or the community. Sterile packs or syringes are opened and not used. Patients or doctors or nurses are kept waiting at clinics or in wards, held up by matters which may be small but are very costly in time. Lights are left on. Irrelevant tests are ordered and performed. And there are many other examples. Under the headings of people (patients and professionals), property, and public funding, make a list of:

- Areas of waste in your own clinical situation.
- How you would change this.
- How, in particular, these affect patient care.

(c) *The cost of investigation*: Much of medical practice is now concerned with the investigation of disease and illness. In general this has been of enormous benefit, the newer tests leading to better diagnosis and better management, but investigations cost money, and there is the additional cost to the patient in terms of time, inconvenience and, in some cases, discomfort. Finally, if investigations are to be performed it is essential that they are used in the management of the patient. Thus, admission to an acute hospital bed to carry out an expensive investigation, which may involve a risk to the patient, must be carefully considered. Ask yourself the following questions and, if you do not know the answer, find it out from your local expert (it will be interesting to see if they know!).

- What is the cost per day of in-patient care in an acute hospital bed?
- What is the current cost of a chest radiograph?
- Can you give a recent example of an unnecessary investigation? Why do you think it was performed?
- Have you seen examples of patients experiencing discomfort in relation to investigations?

Let us suppose that there is a good clinical indication for carrying out an intravenous pyelogram (IVP) in a patient with, for example, evidence of kidney disease, renal stone, etc. It requires a series of abdominal radiographs to be taken and has a very small morbidity and an even smaller mortality associated with it. How would you view using this procedure (remember there is a *good* indication for the test) in the following situations?

- A child with spina bifida
- A pregnant woman
- A 79-year-old man

If your answers to any of the above indicate that you would *not* carry out an IVP, is the reason economic, clinical, or moral?

(d) *The cost of treatment*: Much of medical practice involves the use of treatment − surgical operations, drug treatment, or new methods such as lasers, interleukins, etc. Because there is a finite limit to the resources available it is necessary to make choices. Often we are unaware of the costs of treatment. Take some simple examples of the cost of treatment at 1993 prices.

100 tablets of diazepam 20p
100 tablets of ampicillin £7.12p

100 tablets of ferrous sulphate 45p
1 dose of doxorubicin (anti-cancer drug) £155.00p
1 week of total parenteral nutrition £300.00p
1 hour operating theatre cost £300.00p

There are, therefore, substantial costs associated with all forms of treatment. The use of QALYs has shown that renal transplantation is more cost-effective than dialysis and that coronary artery bypass grafting is a very useful procedure. But the questions are often not simple. Take the 'home' versus 'hospital' argument, for example. In the section on quality of life we looked at the effect on quality of life of the patient and the family of sending the patient home. Look at it now from an economic point of view.

- List the costs of being at home and the costs of being in hospital.
- Include 'indirect' costs of travel, heating, lighting, and food.
- Add the staff costs involved.
- Do these facts in any way change the arguments for and against sending a patient home? Are the arguments you would use moral, economic, or a mixture of both?

Take the story of a boy with a wound in the leg which was told in Chapter 2. Admission might well improve his leg, but at the exclusion of two other patients for routine operations. How would you go about analysing this situation?

1. Consider first the *clinical* reasons for admission. Is it really necessary?
2. Consider the *economic* arguments, the costs of admitting one boy against two others.
3. Consider the *moral* arguments for and against admission.
4. Can these types of argument really be separated?

- A major problem at present for all health care professionals is the provision of care for the elderly. This is a very costly service to run because of the numbers involved. The methods used vary from one part of the country to another, depending on local expertise and resources. Look at the problem from the point of view of QALYs, and try to analyse the various ways in which provision of care could be provided:

Home, hospital, sheltered housing, etc.
Supporting social services required.
Level of medical and nursing care required, etc.

Having done this do you think this kind of analysis would influence your decision the next time you see an elderly patient who wishes to go home?

6. POLITICAL FACTORS IN THE ALLOCATION OF RESOURCES

It is clear that political factors can influence the use of resources. The variations in the provision of care indicate that some special interests are favoured more than others. In addition to the policies of central government there are other political interests which can affect the ways in which health care is provided: local pressure groups, for example, or local charities which may wish to buy a particular piece of equipment for a hospital and thereby create revenue consequences in maintenance or staffing. Look at these examples.

1. Within a major teaching hospital there is a renal dialysis unit. A limited number of machines, nurses, doctors, etc., are available and running costs are also limited. The local patients' group raises £200 000 to buy three new machines and offers them to the hospital. If the hospital *does* accept these machines they will cost an additional £100 000 a year in staff and running costs. In spite of this very generous offer the hospital declines.

- Analyse this situation from an economic and moral point of view.
- Do you agree with the decision?

2. Situated within a major hospital there is a small maternity unit which provides an excellent local service to the community. For

economic reasons, the Health Authority puts forward cogent arguments that a million pounds a year could be saved by closing the hospital and transferring the patients elsewhere. Not surprisingly there is a major outcry locally by the public, patients, and professionals.

- Assuming that the closure *would* save a million pounds *and* that this is essential, look at the arguments for and against closure on economic and moral grounds.
- How much weight would you place on the continuity of care?

3. In a major city there are five accident and emergency departments within a five-mile radius of the city centre, each staffed 24 hours per day. In the interests of economy, and in an attempt to provide a better service for the patient, it is decided to close two of these. The clinical argument is that, with only three departments to staff, a very high level of patient care could be maintained. Local feeling is high, and you are asked, as an outsider, to analyse the economic, clinical, and moral aspects.

- Present a short resume of your analysis.
- Do you think these two units should close?

7. PRIVATE MEDICINE AND THE VOLUNTARY SECTOR

Some aspects of care are provided outside the National Health Service by private hospitals, charitable organizations, and the voluntary sector. They make a valuable contribution to providing care. The development of the purchaser–provider system is described earlier in this chapter and outlines the way in which they can be increasingly involved by providing services to a particular standard and quality. A number of ethical issues arise.

1. The potential problem of a doctor in the NHS spending more time than his or her contract allows on private practice, with knock-on consequences in the Health Service.

2. The importance of patient choice in being able to select the way in which their health care is delivered. It would infringe personal freedom if the right to practise and choose private medicine were removed.

3. There is the potential moral problem in private medicine if treatments or procedures are carried out without proper back-up and facilities.

4. The voluntary sector (e.g. in cancer and AIDS treatment) may put substantial resources into caring for people. It could be argued that the NHS should provide such facilities or that, by adding such substantial resources, priorities are distorted.

Offer some comments:

- How do you view private medicine? How should it fit into the Health Service?
- What role should the voluntary sector play in delivering health care? What are the advantages and disadvantages?

8. CLINICAL FREEDOM

The concept of 'clinical freedom' is an interesting one, in that it has moral, technical and economic overtones. The concept is generally associated with medical practice, though in a wider sense it may apply to all health professional groups. In essence the concept implies: I will do my best for patients or clients referred to me. The decisions I make will be mine and will always be in the best interests of the patient. I will use procedures, equipment, or drugs to this end, regardless of the cost.

There are several important aspects to these statements. The first is that the doctor, or other health care professional, is accountable to himself or herself. The clinical practice which is delivered is determined by the consultant, irrespective of the constraints around him, be these medical, moral, or economic. It is necessary to challenge this assumption and to ask whether or not doctors should have this freedom and, if not, how it should be regulated. Most would agree that professional groups themselves should, by the process of audit, assessment, and monitoring, measure their own performance.

The second implication is one of cost. The concept suggests that a health care professional can use any procedure or drug, no matter what it costs, 'as long as it is in the best interests of the patient'. This aspect too must be questioned. Clearly, there will be instances in which high cost procedures and medication *will* be clinically indicated, but what control should there be over the cost component? In general practice prescription costs are carefully monitored and those who go over an arbitrary limit are asked to justify the expense. This could be a useful model for other professional groups.

- What do you think of the concept of 'clinical freedom'?
- Should it be abandoned?
- How can an effective system of control be introduced?
- Who should make the decisions about what is in the 'best interests of the patient'?

9. THE PUBLIC DIMENSION

Ultimately, it is the public whose opinion is expressed through their duly elected parliamentary representatives who allocate resources. Over the last few years a number of initiatives have been taken, notably in Oregon in the USA, in which public involvement in decision-making has been sought. In general, this can be at the level of the individual patient in enhancing patient choice, or at the macro-level in making decisions about overall resource allocation.

Given that public involvement is important

- How would you go about encouraging it?
- Who would you consider represents the public?

10. CONCLUSION

This chapter has tried to show the very close relationship that exists between moral, clinical, and economic factors in decision-making. In many cases it is not possible to separate them. It is suggested, as has been done several times in this book, that logical analysis of the situation can help to clarify the issues and make judgements and decisions more rational.

Chapter 18

MORAL ASPECTS OF RESEARCH

Research and development are central to the improvement of clinical practice. Without them no progress could be made in treatment, diagnosis, and prevention. Advances in psychological and social research are continually changing the way in which we view patient care. New developments in treatment raise new moral problems.

In a very real sense health care professionals have an obligation to carry out research as part of their function to improve continually the quality of care provided. For this reason, therefore, the ethical issues related to research are directly relevant to all. In addition, there is an increasing recognition that the introduction of a new procedure or treatment, without full evaluation or comparison with existing methods, may result in an ineffective, and possible harmful treatment being used. This relates closely to the outcomes of care and the quality of care provided, both to the individual and the community.

Clinical Audit and Research are sometimes confused, but, while there is an overlap, they serve different functions. Audit is the systematic analysis of equality of clinical care and is based on existing standards and guide-lines. Research looks at new procedures and takes care beyond that currently available. Just as it is important to carry out research so it is necessary, for ethical reasons, for the health care professional to evaluate continually and critically the quality of work. Not to do this may have consequences for the individual.

This chapter deals with a range of issues in relation to research and experimentation.

1. ANIMAL EXPERIMENTATION

In the past many of the developments in health care have been researched initially on animals. Animals may be used for *non-medical* purposes, but this will not be discussed here. In medical research, animals have been used for three main purposes:

1. Testing of new drugs or products.
2. Study of basic mechanisms of body function in health or disease.
3. Testing of hypotheses about physiological or pathological processes.

The argument may be put that animals are living and feeling (sentient) beings and therefore should not in any circumstances be used for experimental purposes. It is argued that it is morally wrong to inflict pain on any living creature even for motives which are of the highest order, such as the search for the cure of a particular disease affecting humans. This is the moral argument, but there is also a scientific argument against the use of animals. It is that because animals are *not* human any results obtained are not applicable to humans anyway and the experiments are therefore worthless.

In reply it can be maintained that animal experimentation has in fact led to an increased understanding of disease processes and of normal body functions; significant theoretical and practical advances have been made using animal models. It is also claimed that the use of animals is the only way to test adequately for side-effects of new drugs or procedures prior to using them in humans.

Those who do use animals in experimental work follow clear guide-lines laid down by the Home Office (in the United Kingdom). These include the use of as few animals as possible; the use of animals for specific purposes only; avoidance of pain or discomfort; proper safeguards for their use.

This section has presented briefly the views for and against the use of animals for research purposes. In answering the following questions try to clarify your own views on the use of animals in research.

- List the advantages and disadvantages of using animals for research.
- Are there any circumstances in which you *would* use animals?
- Are there circumstances in which you would *not* use animals?
- Would the choice of animal used have any bearing on the above, e.g. mouse, rat, cat, dog, or cow? If so, are there moral, rather than scientific, reasons for the choice of animal model?
- Overall, do you think animals should be used for research purposes?

2. CLINICAL TRIALS

In human terms, experimental work is often associated with clinical trials or studies. Such studies are set up, using humans as subjects, to determine the effectiveness of a particular treatment or procedure and to compare it with other forms of treatment. The results may be viewed in relation to cure, length of survival, modification of the disease (e.g. reduction in blood pressure, reduction in tumour mass), side-effects of the treatment, expense, or quality of life. The type of knowledge obtained may therefore be very variable but the overall objective is the improvement of care for the patients, but not necessarily, as we shall see, for the patient on whom the treatment or procedure is being tried.

Clinical trials may be designed in several ways, each with advantages and disadvantages.

1. *Non-randomized trials*: In this instance a treatment is tried on a group of patients without the use of a control group. Such studies, often called pilot studies, are sometimes carried out in the first phase of trying a new procedure, say to assess the toxicity of the treatment. They are also used in rare conditions.

2. *Randomized studies*: In this instance, patients are divided into two (or more) groups. One group has the standard procedure (drug or operation) and the other the new procedure. Patients are allocated to the groups at random. In some instances randomized studies are followed by further studies with matched controls.

3. *Randomized, double-blind studies*: This form of clinical trial involves similar random allocation of patients, and random selection of the treatment, usually a drug, but the doctor assessing and treating the patient does not know which treatment is being used. The information is kept secret until the trial is completed and the code is then broken. This form of study is used particularly where the unbiased views of the doctor or patient are important in assessing the results.

4. *Cross-over studies*: This is a refinement of 2 and 3 above. Following a period of treatment with drug A, the patient is switched to drug B.

What are the scientific and moral problems involved in these kinds of clinical trial or study? From a scientific point of view the study should be so designed as to ask an important question with sufficient patients and resources available for an answer to be obtained in a reasonable period of time. Many studies are poorly designed and are unlikely to achieve an answer. It is essential, therefore, that before any form of clinical trial or study is started, the statistical design of the study itself is carefully scrutinized.

From the moral point of view there are questions which must be asked. Is it ever right to carry out experiments using live human subjects? How are patients informed about such studies, and what kind of consent is sought? How confidential are the results, and how soon would the study be stopped if the results appeared to be useless? What legal redress does the patient have if something goes wrong? Can double-blind studies ever be justified? From the doctor's point of view there is therefore considerable responsibility in conducting a clinical trial, and guidance at a moral level is often based on the 'my mother' principle. The doctor or nurse involved can be invited to consider whether or not his or her own mother could be included in the trial. Is this a procedure you would allow your family to undergo? Although a simple question, it is one which is worth asking in all research work. The trial should also be scrutinized by an ethical committee (see section 4).

The essential problem and dilemma associated with clinical or drug trials and experimentation on human subjects is that, while it is essential to make progress in the understanding of the nature, causation, prevention, and treatment of disease, to do so may involve inflicting harm. For the health care professional this is the dilemma between caring for the individual (the principle of non-maleficence or benevolence) and caring for the good of the majority (the principle of utility). It thus raises once again the important question of which is the more important or how both can be promoted. This problem was first raised in general terms in Chapter 4 and we have encountered it also in our discussion of health economics and in the trainee's dilemma (Chapter 7, section 2).

In the context of clinical trials the dilemmas are created when the health of the individual will not be promoted by the treatment proposed. The use of control groups, which has already been mentioned, is an example of this. Another example is the commonly used technique of giving a placebo. A placebo is a harmless pill or injection which allows an assessment of the effect of 'giving something' to the patient to be compared with active therapy. In many instances, of course, this 'placebo effect' can be beneficial whereas the 'real' drug may be ineffective or even harmful. Hence, the moral problem is not a straightforward one.

It is worth noting that some patients, who are themselves in poor health and unable to contribute any longer to society, voluntarily offer their services for clinical trials or experiments hoping thereby that out of their own poor health some benefits to others may come. This suggests that the key to the moral dilemmas associated with experiments or trials on human subjects lies in the word 'consent'. There is much to be said for this view and we shall now proceed to an analysis of consent.

3. CONSENT

Consent is a concept which is related not just to clinical trials and experimental techniques, but to any relationship between patients or clients and health care professionals. Indeed, we have already referred to it in our discussion of the consultation. To bring out the centrality of the concept of consent in health care let us review the situation of the patient who is *not* part of a clinical trial as this is the normal state of affairs for the majority of patients. The assumptions in the consultation are:

(1) that the doctor knows the possibilities of treatment; and
(2) that he has the skills to carry them out.

In this context consent is just as important as it is in a full-blown clinical trial. Take the patient who comes to his general practitioner with a minor infection for which an antibiotic is prescribed. This, in a sense, is a clinical trial and as such the questions of disclosure of information and of consent must also be raised even though it is in a relatively minor situation. Turn now to the hospital context.

In a hospital context consent is involved in all types of contact between patients and professionals. For example, consent would be required:

Before bed-bathing a patient.
Before taking a blood sample.
Before clinical examination, etc.

Consent is a necessary part of any health care relationship and requires careful analysis. Let us begin the analysis by offering a definition of consent.

(a) *Definition of consent*: Consent may be defined as the granting to someone the permission to do something he would not have the right to do without such permission. In clinical practice the word 'consent' often has a series of adjectives associated with it, including implied, informed, voluntary, competent, valid.

We shall shortly go on to analyse these terms, but first let us consider why there is a moral need for consent and later, in (h), consider whether asking for consent can ever be harmful.

(b) *Need for consent* (See Chapter 4, section 2): There are several reasons why consent is morally necessary for health care intervention. These reasons involve, in different ways, all the basic moral principles of health care which we outlined in Chapter 4.

1. *Respect for individual autonomy.* The individual with his rights of self-determination and self-government is considered to be the most important factor in the moral requirement for consent. The principle of autonomy is the relevant one here.

2. *Protection of patients and subjects.* Consent allows the patient or subject to say 'no', and enables him to be aware of the risks of the procedure or treatment. The principle of non-maleficence with its positive side of benevolence is relevant to this justification.

3. *Avoidance of fraud or duress.* The patient in a consultation is very vulnerable, especially if he or she is ill. It is not difficult in these circumstances to persuade patients to undergo a particular type of procedure. Once again the principle of non-maleficence is relevant, and also the principle of justice − it may be unfair to persuade a patient to undergo a certain treatment or to take part in a certain trial.

4. *The use of self-audit by professionals.* To ask for consent means that the professional has recognized that a problem exists and can then scrutinize his own motives in wishing to suggest the treatment or procedure. The self-referring principle of self-development or integrity is the one relevant here.

5. *Promotion of rational decisions.* The use of self-audit should begin to make the doctor or nurse or other professional think more clearly about decisions. This is again the principle of

self-development, but also the principle of utility, for clearly the consequences for the majority of patients are improved if health care professionals are obliged to explain and justify their treatments to their patients.

6. *Promotion of public and social values*. By raising the general issues of consent, health care professionals involve the general public in decision-making and educate public attitudes. This is clearly a justification expressed in terms of the principle of utility.

It should be clear from these reasons that consent is a very important moral concept for everyday clinical practice, and that it is related to all the basic principles of health care. Yet the most fundamental justification in terms of the philosophy of this book must be the first. Unless an autonomous person consents to treatment the health care professional has no right to intervene at all — what he does may constitute an assault from the moral and sometimes even from the legal point of view. This can be difficult for benevolent and caring professionals to accept, and indeed as we shall see in paragraph (h) there can be difficult cases.

(c) *Implied consent*: It is sometimes said that for practical purposes consent can be assumed. This is often called 'implied consent'. The patient comes to the doctor or dentist wishing advice and help. Implicit in this is the assumption that confidential information can be shared, physical examinations carried out, and treatment or action taken without asking formally for consent. This attitude could certainly be questioned; there are surely limits to what a patient can be thought to have consented to by having a consultation.

(d) *Informed consent*: Much of the discussion on the subject of consent concerns the analysis of the term 'informed', and many questions have been raised about its definition. For example:

Is it possible for a 'lay' person to be fully informed?
Does all the information about possible side-effects have to be communicated?

What if the doctor does not know all about the possible side-effects?

(e) *Voluntary consent*: There is no difficulty about understanding what this means — the patient consents of his own free will and is not coerced or pressured to agree. The difficulty lies in determining whether in given cases the consent is really voluntary. A person who suspects or knows that his/her prognosis is not good is likely to agree to anything and the distinctions between treatment, therapeutic research, and non-therapeutic research may not mean much. It is therefore a real question whether in many cases there is any possibility of voluntary consent. The patient may be too vulnerable to refuse.

(f) *Competence to consent*: In this context competence means the ability to comprehend the information given. This places children, psychiatrically disturbed individuals, and unconscious patients in a difficult situation, and this has already been discussed in Chapter 5.

(g) *Valid consent*: This ideally contains the following elements:

Information
1. Disclosure of information. (But how much and how soon?)
2. Comprehension of the information. (Is it really understood?)

Consent
1. This should be voluntary. (Can it ever be fully voluntary?)
2. The patient should be 'competent' to consent. (But there are borderline cases.)

In the following examples think carefully about consent and analyse the situation carefully before answering the question. It is recognized that further information may be required to give an answer. If this is the case, list the kind of information you would need.

1. A 42-year-old man presents to his general practitioner with a cough and some breathlessness and the diagnosis of chronic

bronchitis is made. An antibiotic is prescribed which has the following side-effects:

5 per cent chance of diarrhoea.

1 per cent chance of a drug sensitivity reaction.

- What kind of consent should be sought before commencing this drug?
- Would this fit into the category of 'implied consent'?

2. A 50-year-old woman is referred to a hospital consultant with a history of lower abdominal pain and some disturbance of bowel function.

A physical examination is required including abdominal examination, rectal and vaginal examination.

- What kind of consent is required? Verbal? Written?

3. A diagnostic procedure known as lymphangiography is very useful in investigating some forms of disease, notably cancer. Dye is injected into the foot and radiographs are taken subsequent to this over the following 24 hours. The abdominal lymph nodes are outlined. the following information is available:

The patient requires admission for 24 hours.

There is a 1 per cent chance of wound infection.

There is a 0.5 per cent chance of serious breathlessness.

There is a 0.05 per cent chance of death.

- Describe the consent required. Specifically decide on whether or not the patient should be told of the risk of death.
- What if the diagnosis is in doubt and the patient has not yet been informed of the nature of the disease?

4. A 60-year-old man is dying from lung cancer. He has back pain which is not well controlled by analgesics (pain-killers) and he has had radio-therapy. A new pain-killer has been developed and you wish to try it on this patient.

- Outline the consent required.

5. An 18-year-old man has been seriously injured in a road accident. He is on a ventilator and has been diagnosed as being

'brain-dead' using the appropriate criteria (see Chapter 16, section 1). You wish to obtain consent for the removal of his kidneys.

- Whom do you ask?
- Draw up a consent document.

(h) *Can consent be harmful?* Throughout this discussion it has been assumed that asking for consent to a particular procedure is always morally required, and that seeking it is therefore always justifiable. But we indicated at the end of (a) that in some circumstances seeking consent may be harmful. Suppose, for example, that a series of options about treatment is given to the patient, but that treatment A is recommended. Suppose further that the patient does *not* consent to this, but requests treatment B. This is then duly given, but fails. In these circumstances feelings of guilt and anger may become apparent in the patient and doctor. Consent and choice are closely related and while the positive aspects of both can be readily seen the potential negative aspects must always be remembered. The tension here is between respect for the autonomy of the patient, even if he is making what the health care professional regards as a misguided decision, and the desire of the professional, governed by the principle of benevolence, to help the patient.

- Do you think that obtaining consent is always required?

(i) *Ways of thinking about consent*: Consent may be viewed in three broad ways as:

1. A legally restrictive device designed to protect the patient from harm and to preserve his or her autonomy. This could be considered as a very narrow view of consent.
2. A legal protection for the professional if things go wrong. Again, this could seem narrow.
3. An extension of the patient–doctor, patient–professional relationship, one built on trust in which any form of consent, informed, voluntary, written, etc., is seen as a natural extension of the trust established.

● Consider these ways of thinking about consent. Which do you prefer?

4. THE ROLE OF ETHICAL COMMITTEES

Most hospitals now have Ethical Committees to review research proposals submitted by the professional staff. These committees comprise representatives of the medical staff, nursing staff, and other professional groups and lay representatives. They therefore act in two ways — first, as a method of peer review by professionals, and second, as a technique for lay review. Such committees therefore perform an increasingly important function.

● Are there ethical committees at the hospital to which you are attached?
● If so, who are the members, how often do they meet and what questions do they address?

5. INTERPROFESSIONAL CONFLICTS

Research is an area in which the potential for conflict between professional groups can certainly occur. This is often related to a misunderstanding of the nature of the research and poor communication between the groups concerned. The nursing staff may feel that the research appears more important than the patients' comfort. Yet how are new advances to be made?

These conflicts raise the important question as to whether research is always justifiable. While this might well be considered to be a predominantly medical problem at present, the increasing involvement of other groups, such as nurses, dietitians, psychologists, and social workers in research, means that this may not always be so. Research projects can alter relationships within the team and divided loyalties can occur. (See also section 10.)

- Can you draw up criteria for justifiable research in health care?

6. NURSING RESEARCH

Research into aspects of nursing is developing rapidly and bringing with it its own moral problems. Nurses are used to dealing with immediate problems and solving them. To stand back and just observe can be difficult. For example, it may not be easy for a 'research nurse' simply to study a nursing procedure and not take part or assist in it. This is especially the case if the nurse being studied is not carrying out the procedure in a satisfactory way. How far can the 'research nurse' intervene? The presence of the research nurse will modify the situation of course and may change the practice.

A number of nursing projects are concerned with assessing the psychological state of the patient after a particular procedure or treatment. Such projects require great sensitivity on behalf of the research worker. Studying bereavement problems can raise issues with relatives which they might not have wished to discuss. Research into the value of counselling raises similar moral issues. There may be positive harm in such studies unless they are carefully prepared and carried out. Suppose that, as above, the counselling appears misguided. Does the nurse then intervene and in so doing alter the study?

Many of the observational research projects do involve an invasion of privacy, both for the patient and the nurse. Just as in research carried out by doctors on medical problems, questions of competence and caring will be raised. The special problem of 'control' groups also needs to be discussed. As in many studies looking at aspects of care, the group of patients under investigation often gets better care than the 'non-study' group. One only has to think of the inequality of distribution of clinical nurse specialists to realize that this occurs. As part of the study it is often essential that there is a 'control' group.

- What responsibility would you as a research nurse have for the control group?

At present the nursing profession sees itself as 'the patient's advocate' in relation to research. If nursing research develops, as indeed is likely, then perhaps the doctor or the social worker will act in the capacity of 'advocate' to ensure that the patient is protected from the intrusions of research.

Much of the potential 'conflict' in research is related to poor communication about the aims of the research project and the responsibility of the team. This is a theme which has been taken up in Chapter 12, section 4.

● What are the special moral problems of nursing, as distinct from medical, research?

7. EPIDEMIOLOGICAL RESEARCH

So far, the discussion has been based on research problems directly affecting individual patients. There are, however, other aspects of research which deal with populations of patients. These studies, generally of an epidemiological nature, involve surveys of disease, personal characteristics, social information, etc. They are frequently carried out by interview techniques or by using questionnaires. A great deal of sensitive information may be collected in this way. By standard computing techniques it is possible to link one set of records with another if the patient or individual can be identified. The confidentiality of such data is therefore of paramount importance.

Important ethical issues arise from survey research and epidemiological work. For example, during an anonymous survey of patients for a particular disease to estimate the incidence or prevalence of the illness, it may be that individuals who do not know they have the disease are identified. Because the survey is anonymous the individual will therefore not be informed. A second issue arises related to the identification of an individual with an unknown problem; for example, a raised blood pressure or cholesterol level, which is then recorded in the medical notes. As part of the research procedure this is then identified as a clinical issue that may have consequences for that individual in relation to other aspects of their life, such as insurance. It may also mean that the individual is then given treatment which in itself may have consequences. Thus, in the planning of epidemiological and survey research these broader ethical implications must be considered.

8. HEALTH CARE RESEARCH

There is increasing interest in studying the Health Service itself, the quality of care provided and the cost-effectiveness of the service. This involves studying in detail the work of individual doctors, nurses, social workers, etc. It requires measures of effectiveness. The moral problems here involve situations where care may be found to be substandard or deficient, or where inadequate resources are being provided to cover a particular health need. For example, an investigation of the work of a clinical unit might indicate that additional nursing staff are required to carry out the functions in an effective way. The research team would then have to deal with moral problems involved in these findings. This raises the general question of the role of the research worker and this will now be discussed in more detail.

9. MORAL RESPONSIBILITIES OF THE
RESEARCH WORKER

Much of the literature in the field of moral aspects of research deals with the rights of patients, but those carrying out research may also have moral problems. For example, suppose a new procedure is found to be harmful, rather than helpful. How soon should this information be made public and what responsibilities are there to the patients under study? This is just one example of a number of possible problems. Here are a few others. Consider them in detail and how you would respond if you were a member of the research team.

- During the course of a laboratory research project you become concerned that one of the research assistants is not providing accurate results and may even be 'fiddling' them. What would you do?

- In a project designed to study the psychological impact of treatment on patient care it is noted that one of the research workers is quite unsuited to being part of the study. She is upsetting patients and there is now general resistance within the clinical team to continuing with the project. Would you call a team meeting to discuss the approach to the patients? Ask the worker to leave? Try to stop the project?

- An epidemiological survey of infective problems in hospitals in a Health Region shows that one hospital has a particularly bad record. The incidence of gastrointestinal infection is five times that of other hospitals. Who should be informed?

- In the course of carrying out a survey of medication given to elderly patients it becomes clear that there is a higher mortality among a group given two specific drugs in combination. Do you wait until your results are published before doing anything?

- You have been asked to review the services for a particular specialty in your area (e.g. obstetrics, accident, and emergency medicine). Your research indicates clearly that one hospital has spare capacity, and by re-arrangement it could well be closed. Consider the moral, as opposed to the economic, implications of this decision.

Consideration of the above problems should reveal that the research workers cannot morally detach themselves from the results of their projects. Those involved in research must therefore take responsibility for the moral implication both of the process (how the research is carried out) and the outcome (the results of the project).

10. PUBLISH OR PERISH

There is increasing pressure on health care professionals to publish the results of research work. In medicine in particular it would be very unusual for a senior appointment to be made without the individual having a significant number of publications. In some ways this is laudable. The ability to publish the results of research work indicates an ability to finish a project and write it up. It is also an indication of the commitment to teaching, research and development of the subject. Several moral problems can arise however in this quest for publications.

1. Patients may be seen as objects which will ensure promotion.
2. The quality of the research may be poor.
3. A research project may be submitted to several journals with minor modifications massaged by the word processor. There will therefore be several publications with the titles changed.

These examples, once again, highlight the moral responsibilities of those taking part in research programmes.

11. THE USE OF VOLUNTEERS IN RESEARCH

For some purposes it is considered necessary to use normal human volunteers for research purposes. There are, however, potential dangers to this approach, particularly if the procedure is invasive or associated with potentially harmful side-effects. A particularly vulnerable group are medical students who may be asked to take part as normal subjects in a research project. Recently there have been serious consequences of this.

● If you were asked to take part in a new drug trial as a 'normal control' what information would you require before you said yes or no? Would you be prepared to take part in such trials under any circumstances? How would you react if you were offered a large sum of money by a drug company as an inducement?

12. FUNDING OF RESEARCH

As we have seen in Chapter 17 there is a finite amount of money available to provide for health care. For this reason choices have to be made — it is exactly the same in relation to the funding of research; priorities have to be worked out. There is a basic conflict, for example, between the need to fund basic research which might lead to fundamental changes in our understanding of disease, and health care research which is primarily directed at patient care. If research funding is limited, difficult choices have to be made — for example, to support research into *in vitro* fertilization and genetically inherited disease, or into the problems of *dementia* in the elderly. Both are important, but there is insufficient money to go round.

- Draw up a list of priorities for funding in basic research and health care research.

A further moral problem which is related to funding is the *source* of money.

- Is it morally acceptable to accept money from the pharmaceutical industry to carry out research on their products?
- What about money from the tobacco industry? Should it be accepted?

Much of the research funded in the United Kingdom comes from charitable sources. Without this a great deal of the research just could not be done.

- What obligation does the state have to support research?

13. CONCLUSION

Looking back over the last 10 years there have been important developments in medical research. 'New' diseases have been discovered such as AIDS and Legionnaires' disease and new treatments developed. These include coronary artery bypass surgery, transplantation of liver, heart, and bone marrow, *in vitro* fertilization, surrogate motherhood, prenatal diagnosis, genetic engineering, and many others. What is clear is that over the next 10 years more advances will be made and, as professional health care workers, we must be ready to meet the challenges they pose. If the next 10 years are as interesting from a moral point of view as the past 10 years, then there will be plenty to discuss.

Chapter 19

QUALITY IN HEALTH CARE

There is no doubt that quality is a central issue in health care at present. Indeed, it could be said that quality is at the heart of clinical practice. The concept, however, is not new and can be viewed as part of the long tradition of professional practice. Recently, targets and quantitative aspects have been introduced into the measurement of quality − for example, in relation to immunization − formalizing what has been until now a fairly subjective approach. It is also an issue which is part of professional development and education and is related to clinical audit, accreditation, standards, guide-lines, and protocols.

1. DEFINITION OF QUALITY

The topic of quality raises a series of difficult questions including what does quality mean, how can it be measured, and who should measure it? The literature is full of definitions, and the following, though not entirely original, tries to encapsulate some important components.

Quality is a concept which describes in both quantitative and qualitative terms the level of care or services provided. Quality as a concept therefore has two components. The first is quantitative and measurable, the second is qualitative, though assessable, and associated with value judgements. Quality is a relative not an absolute concept.

Quality is not therefore an analysis of activity. In describing the quality of a service it must always be compared to something else − either a similar activity or the same activity measured at another time. It also implies measurable consistency over time. Thus quality, as a relative concept, can always be improved, and that is at the heart of all quality initiatives, the process of continual improvement.

Quality can be related to the achievement of specific aims, objectives, standards, and targets. Those standards should not be seen as fixed, as they will inevitably change as medical advances arise and improve the outcome of care.

As quality of care is a multidimensional issue, how can the quality of care provided by doctors or other health care professionals be measured? The following suggestions are made to stimulate discussion and to raise a further question as to who should measure quality. Thus, quality of medical care, as an example, could be seen to comprise:

- Knowledge, technical skill, and competence
- Professional standards, including ethical issues
- Attitudes and behaviour, including communication skills
- Managerial functions, including the ability to work within resources
- Teaching, audit, and research.

There is considerable overlap between these headings, but for each it is possible to determine how, and who, should measure performance. For example, it might be reasonable that the first of these − knowledge, technical skills, and competence − would be assessed by doctors, but that most of the others could be assessed by other professionals, managers, and the public, as well as by doctors. Objective as well as subjective assessments are required.

This raises the general issue of Total Quality Management and Continuous Quality Improvement. Both of these initiatives are being developed within the National Health Service. They build on two crucial principles which are well-established elsewhere and should be equally familiar to those in the health service.

1. Do things right first time.
2. Work for continual improvement.

2. OUTCOME OF HEALTH CARE

An outcome of health care might be said to be the effect on the patient, family, and community as the end result of one or more episodes of care provided over a period of time for an individual. Episodes of care may be judged objectively and subjectively by that individual, the community, and the professional staff involved. The outcome must be related to the objectives of care set by the patient and staff at the start of the episode. Outcomes are important because they form the basis of decision-making, and hence resource allocation, and identify areas requiring more work. This definition emphasizes the importance of time in determining outcome and, in addition to objective measures, the need for subjective evaluation and value judgements. It also places some onus on the community to be involved in assessing outcome, as its measurement will be one factor in determining the need for resources. Finally, it makes the point that patients should be involved in setting the objectives of their care at the start of the process.

- What factors do you consider influence the outcome of health care?
- How far do you think that the level of resources available influences outcome?

3. OUTCOMES IN A WIDER CONTEXT

Outcomes are generally considered in relation to the effect on the individual patient. But three others matters need to be considered. The first relates to the role of professional staff in measurement. They have a crucial role in assessment of outcome, and, indeed, this process should be part of routine practice. However, there may be differences between what a patient or relative and a doctor thinks of as a 'good' outcome.

These differences should be recognized and analysed. They can be the beginning of greater insight into 'outcomes' for staff, relatives, and patients. Thus, what patients and families think of as 'quality' and their response to existing services need to be carefully considered.

The second issue relates to quality, outcomes, and the community. Ultimately it is the public, through a series of processes, who determine the resources for health care. It is important therefore that the public, as citizens, as well as potential patients, are informed and involved in what outcomes and quality mean and that this dialogue is seen to be part of the ongoing process of continually improving the service. This represents a further challenge to doctors in communicating to the public the nature of the issues concerned and the standards of care which can be expected.

Assessment of outcomes is very complicated. It requires an ability to measure baseline and end-point states, whether in relation to health, reassurance, satisfaction, or other effects. Measurement of health, which, as already mentioned, includes not only disease states but also function and patients' perceptions of well-being, is in itself complicated. But outcomes go beyond just measurement of change from baseline to end-point. For such change to reflect quality of care we have to be able to demonstrate that it was actually a result of that particular care. Demonstrating a change in health status, for example, requires teasing out the effect of that care from all other possible influences on health.

The third issue relates to implications for managers. Managers, including those doctors who manage resources, need to be aware of the consequences of searching for quality and continually improving the service. All concerned are on the same side and should be working as a team towards better patient care.

- Give an example of how the outcome for a patient may differ from that of the professional.
- Take an example of a clinical problem you were associated with recently. How would you measure the quality of the care?

4. GUIDE-LINES, PROTOCOLS, AND STANDARDS

It is important that these three terms are not confused. Protocols relate to specific illnesses and are generally tightly written; deviation from them is unusual. Guide-lines are more flexible and more general. Standards indicate the overall objective of management and may be achieved by using guide-lines and protocols.

In general, it seems to be a good idea to ensure that methods of patient management are written down and agreed. The educational value of doing this is, in fact, considerable. There are, however, some problems. The first is the obvious problem of the patient whose management does not quite fit into a particular protocol, or who, for perfectly good reasons, does not wish to agree to the proposed management − that is,the patient choice factor. The second is the issue of clinical freedom and the need to be able to improve current best practice and to carry out research and development. The third is in some ways more serious and refers to possible legal constraints if protocols or guide-lines are not adhered to. Each of these issues can be overcome, and the whole process could be kept within the professional sphere with one important proviso − namely, the ability to deal with doctors or other professionals who do not perform to an adequate standard. Professional competence will be discussed in more detail later. Finally, there is the issue of resources, an important element in the development of standards.

- What do you consider to be the main ethical issues in using standards and guide-lines in clinical practice?
- Who should set clinical standards? Patients, professionals, managers, or politicians?

A further function of writing down standards is that they can then be communicated to others, including patients and the public at large, who have a right to know what to expect of treatment and its outcome, and to assume that their clinical team is using up-to-date methods of treatment. Finally, there is a real educational value in communicating with other staff about the standards to be adopted and delivered. The audit process and the development of guide-lines are thus powerful aspects of continuing education.

5. COMPETENCE AND PERFORMANCE REVIEW

Competence is an issue central to quality. It concerns standards of care and the knowledge, skills, and attitudes which doctors and other health professionals should possess at different periods in their career. Thus, it should be possible to distinguish between a house officer and consultant in terms of performance and competence. The assessment of competence is an important activity and relates the performance of an individual doctor to a given set of criteria. In general, it is carried out by other doctors and based on comparisons with others in similar specialties and grades. As discussed earlier, there is of course no reason why the assessment should be the responsibility of doctors. Others, including nursing staff, managers, and patients have a role in the process. Indeed, it might be claimed that they could be more objective than doctors.

The criteria by which an assessment of competence is based can be derived in various ways. The simplest is to compare the activity and the outcome of care provided by an individual doctor with that provided by a range of other doctors. This can be done by observation and by objective measurement of evidence of activity and outcome, such as results of treatment, scrutiny of case-sheets, participation in clinical trials, and the results of audit. The results may be compared with others working in the same geographical area, or in other parts of the country, or abroad. From such experiences it becomes possible to identify the criteria required of the competent doctor.

Another way of developing such criteria is to use the process of critical incident analysis. Such a process analyses the results of asking large numbers of doctors in a particular specialty what are the areas of particular difficulty or importance and which are easier to deliver. From this an assessment can be made of those areas, or 'competencies' which are required to deliver a proper level of service. These can then be evaluated in the individual doctor.

Once a doctor has been designated as 'competent', perhaps at the end of the period of postgraduate training, the next question which arises is whether or not he or she should at regular intervals undergo periodic 'accreditation'. In an ideal world, continuing medical education would be the way in which doctors kept up to date. For various reasons this may not be sufficient in itself, without some incentive to continue to learn. It is for this reason that several medical organizations in different parts of the world have used some form of re-accreditation process. In general, this involves a formal assessment of work-load, outcome, and audit of clinical work, and education experience, on a regular basis − for example, every five or ten years. This is not the norm, but several specialist societies and colleges are discussing its implementation. There is an ethical obligation for doctors to ensure that the management of an individual patient is both competent and up to date. This is the least that patients can expect.

- In your own professional group, and at your current level of experience, list a series of ways by which competence might be assessed.
- How should health care professionals who are not competent be dealt with? Should professional self-regulations be the main method of controlling professional competence?
- How would you react to regular (5−7 years) competency assessments once you have reached your career grade?

6. CONCLUSIONS

Creating a climate and culture of quality and excellence should be part of professional education. This emphasizes the need to create an atmosphere, an ethos, a social context, in which certain standards of behaviour and professionalism are seen to be built into the education and training in medical schools, and through postgraduate training and continuing medical education.

The challenges, repeatedly emphasized, are there to be seized. In the interests of continually improving the quality of the service it is essential that doctors and other professional groups pick up the challenge and take part in leading the process of change and improvement.

Chapter 20

CODES OF ETHICS

1. LIMITATIONS OF CODES

In our Introduction we distinguished three senses of the term 'ethics': moral philosophy, morality and codes of professional procedures. Having offered discussions under the first two headings we come finally to codes. Indeed, no book on the morality of health care is complete without the inclusion of some of the traditional codes of ethics. From the earliest beginnings of health care there has been an awareness of its moral dimension, and until the 1960s this awareness was expressed almost exclusively in codes of ethics. The reasons for this were that there existed a consensus within the professions as to their values, there was no challenge to those from the general public and little by way of economic constraint from governments. In view of this professional, public, and political consensus it seemed adequate that the ethics of health care should be expressed in deontological form, in other words in a series of 'do's' and 'don'ts'. And indeed it is still worthwhile for every health care professional to be aware of the codes applying to his/her own profession. Nevertheless, it will be clear from what we have said in this book that codes of ethics have limitations and these we shall now discuss.

1. They suggest to professionals that 'ethics' is somehow distinct from the rest of morality. Our position, on the other hand, is that whereas moral problems may crop up more frequently in health care than in some other spheres of life, moral

principles are the same for all of us. Another way of looking at the same point is this. Codes suggest that the professional is *given* his ethics − perhaps even literally given them in a handbook − whereas it is at least as true that the professional *brings with him* his own individual values to his professional life. We have stressed the importance of the individual's having his own values, being aware of them and being willing to change them conscientiously in the light of changing facts.

2. Whereas any profession must lay down *rules* or *duties* for its members (it must have its deontology), there are many aspects of health care which are not expressible in rules. For example, we have discussed the importance of cultivating certain *attitudes*, such as compassion, which are not wholly reducible to rules.

3. Codes tend to be exclusive to *one* profession, whereas we have argued that health care is best delivered by *teams*. And just as codes do not stress the importance of teams so they assume

4. an exclusive professional−patient relationship; the individual professional must do the best he can for the individual patient. But this is to ignore the pressing importance of the *economic side* to health care. We have emphasized the importance of economics in several sections of our book.

5. As we have said, codes assume a consensus on values both within the professions and their public. But it is doubtful whether this still exists on many important questions. The public is now better educated than ever before on health care, is better informed on legal rights, and in general is consumer-conscious. A consequence of this is that patients increasingly demand that health care should be delivered in terms of their own values rather than those of the professions. A good example of this, as we have seen, is in maternity services. To the extent, then, that professions are now expected to work *through* the community rather than *on* it, the position of codes of ethics has shifted from the centre of professional life to the margins.

Nevertheless, there can be contexts in which professions must assert the simple and basic rules of their codes of ethics. For example, the role of some Soviet psychiatrists in their treatment of dissidents seemed to ignore basic rules. Again, the rule of confidentiality can be threatened by legal or political pressure. It is, therefore, important that professions should have codes with which to defend themselves against the wrong sort of political interference. Indeed, over the last decade codes of professional ethics have proliferated rapidly. All health care professionals now have their own code, and it is almost part of the status of being a professional that such codes are written. We have included here five codes of ethics to illustrate certain principles used in the construction of codes. Inevitably many codes or declarations have not been included and the reader is referred to other sources for this information.

2. THE OATH OF HIPPOCRATES

This is perhaps the oldest of the codes of ethics used, and yet it raises many contemporary issues. The importance of teaching and learning, the good of patients and the avoidance of harm, the problems of abortion, the need to know one's limitations, professional conduct and confidentiality are all stressed.

The Oath of Hippocrates

I swear by Apollo the physician, and Aesculapius, and Health, and All-heal, and all the gods and goddesses, that, according to my ability and judgement, I will keep this Oath and this stipulation—to reckon him who taught me this Art equally dear to me as my parents, to share my substance with him, and relieve his necessities if required; to look upon his offspring on the same footing as my own brothers, and to teach them this art, if they shall wish to learn it, without fee or stipulation; and that by precept, lecture, and every other mode of instruction, I will impart a knowledge of the Art to my own sons, and those of my teachers, and to disciples bound by a stipulation and oath according to the law of medicine, but to none others. I will follow that system or regimen which, according to my ability and judgement, I consider for the benefit of my patients, and abstain from whatever is deleterious and mischievous. I will give no deadly medicine to any one if asked, not suggest any such counsel; and in like manner I will not give to a woman a pessary to produce abortion. With purity and with holiness I will pass my life and practise my Art. I will not cut persons laboring under the stone, but will leave this to be done by men who are practitioners of this work.

Into whatever houses I enter, I will go into them for the benefit of the sick, and will abstain from every voluntary act of mischief and corruption; and, further, from the seduction of females or males, of freemen and slaves. Whatever, in connection with my professional practice or not in connection with it, I see or hear in the life of men, which ought not to be spoken of abroad, I will not divulge, as reckoning that all such should be kept secret. While I continue to keep this Oath unviolated, may it be granted to me to enjoy life and the practice of the Art, respected by all men, in all times! But should I trespass and violate this Oath, may the reverse be my lot!

- As a medical student today are you still able to subscribe to this oath?

3. THE DECLARATION OF GENEVA

This is the Code of the World Medical Association (1968). It is shorter than the Hippocratic Oath. It emphasizes that the first consideration of the doctor is the health of the patient. It recognizes respect for human life, but also raises political and social issues.

The World Medical Association
Declaration of Geneva

Physician's Oath
At the time of being admitted as a member of the medical profession:
I solemnly pledge myself to consecrate my life to the service of humanity;
I will give to my teachers the respect and gratitude which is their due;
I will practise my profession with conscience and dignity;
the health of my patient will be my first consideration;
I will maintain by all the means in my power, the honor and the noble traditions of the medical profession;
my colleagues will be my brothers.

(Reprinted by permission.)

- Do you find this more or less satisfactory than the Hippocratic Oath? (See above.)

● If you are not a doctor or medical student, how do you re
to these codes?

4. THE CODE OF PROFESSIONAL CONDUCT FOR THE NURSE, MIDWIFE, AND HEALTH VISITOR

This code, published by the United Kingdom Central Council for Nursing, Midwifery and Health Visiting is an example of a nursing code of ethics. It stresses the importance of the well-being of the patient, and the ability to work in a collaborative and co-operative manner with other health care professionals. It emphasizes the importance of the patient's own customs, values, and spiritual beliefs. It introduced the question of concern for professional colleagues, and specifically mentions the need to refuse gifts which might be interpreted as giving preferential treatment. The commercial problems of being a nurse are also raised.

Codes of Professional Conduct for the Nurse, Midwife and Health Visitor

Each registered nurse, midwife and health visitor shall act, at all times, in such a manner as to justify public trust and confidence, to uphold and enhance the good standing and reputation of the profession, to serve the interests of society, and above all to safeguard the interests of individual patients and clients.

Each registered nurse, midwife and health visitor is accountable for his or her practice, and, in the exercise of professional accountability shall:

1. Act always in such a way as to promote and safeguard the well being and interests of patients/clients.

2. Ensure that no action or omission on his/her part or within his/her sphere of influence is detrimental to the condition of safety of patients/clients.

3. Take every reasonable opportunity to maintain and improve professional knowledge and competence.

4. Acknowledge any limitations of competence and refuse in such cases to accept delegated functions without first having received instruction in regard to those functions and having been assessed as competent.

5. Work in a collaborative and co-operative manner with other health care professionals and recognise and respect their particular contributions within the health care team.

6. Take account of the customs, values and spiritual beliefs of patients/clients.

7. Make known to an appropriate person or authority any conscientious objection which may be relevant to professional practice.

8. Avoid any abuse of the privileged relationship which exists with patients/clients and of the privileged access allowed to their property, residence or workplace.

9. Respect confidential information obtained in the course of professional practice and refrain from disclosing such information without the consent of the patient/client, or a person entitled to act on his/her behalf, except where disclosure is required by law or by the order of a court or is necessary in the public interest.

10. Have regard to the environment of care and its physical, psychological and social effects on patients/clients, and also to the adequacy of resources, and make known to appropriate persons or authorities any circumstances which could place patients/clients in jeopardy or which militate against safe standards of practice.

11. Have regard to the workload of and the pressures on professional colleagues and subordinates and take appropriate action if these are seen to be such as to constitute abuse of the individual practitioner and/or to jeopardise safe standards of practice.

12. In the context of the individual's own knowledge, experience, and sphere of authority, assist peers and subordinates to develop professional competence in accordance with their needs.

13. Refuse to accept any gift, favour or hospitality which might be interpreted as seeking to exert undue influence to obtain preferential consideration.

14. Avoid the use of professional qualifications in the promotion of commercial products in order not to compromise the independence of professional judgement on which patients/clients rely.

(Reprinted by permission.)

- If you are a nurse, or training to be one, could you subscribe to the above code? How does it compare with the Hippocratic Oath?

5. PATIENTS' RIGHTS

Throughout this book we have emphasized the rights of patients. The American Hospital Association has codified this as a Bill of Rights. It considers confidentiality, respect, information provision and consent. It raises matters such as the right to inspect the bill after treatment, where payment is required.

American Hospital Association
A Patient's Bill of Rights

The American Hospital Association presents a Patient's Bill of Rights with the expectation that observance of these rights will contribute to more effective patient care and greater satisfaction for the patient, his physician, and the hospital organization. Further, the Association presents these rights in the expectation that they will be supported by the hospital on behalf of its patients, as an integral part of the healing process. It is recognized that a personal relationship between the physician and the patient is essential for the provision of proper medical care. The traditional physician-patient relationship takes on a new dimension when care is rendered within an organizational structure. Legal precedent has established that the institution itself also has a responsibility to the patient. It is in recognition of these factors that these rights are affirmed.

1. The patient has the right to considerate and respectful care.

2. The patient has the right to obtain from his physician the complete current information concerning his diagnosis, treatment, and prognosis in terms the patient can be reasonably expected to understand. When it is not medically advisable to give such information to the patient, the information should be made available to an appropriate person on his behalf. He has the right to know, by name, the physician responsible for co-ordinating his care.

3. The patient has the right to receive from his physician information necessary to give informed consent prior to the start of any procedure and/or treatment. Except in emergencies, such information for informed consent should include but not necessarily be limited to the specific procedure and/or treatment, the medically significant risks involved, and the probable duration of incapacitation. Where medically significant alternatives for care or treatment exist, or when the patient requests information concerning medical alternatives, the patient has the right to such information. The

patient also has the right to know the name of the person responsible for the procedures and/or treatment.

4. The patient has the right to refuse treatment to the extent permitted by the law and to be informed of the medical consequences of his action.

5. The patient has the right to every consideration of his privacy concerning his own medical care program. Case discussion, consultation, examination, and treatment are confidential and should be conducted discretely. Those not directly involved in his care must have the permission of the patient to be present.

6. The patient has the right to expect that all communications and records pertaining to his care should be treated as confidential.

7. The patient has the right to expect that within its capacity a hospital must make reasonable response to the request of a patient for services. The hospital must provide evaluation, service, and/or referral as indicated by the urgency of the case. When medically permissible, the patient may be transferred to another facility only after he has received complete information and explanation concerning the needs for and alternatives to such a transfer. The institution to which the patient is to be transferred must first have accepted the patient for transfer.

8. The patient has the right to obtain information as to any relationship of his hospital to other health care and educational institutions insofar as his care is concerned. The patient has the right to obtain information as to the existence of any professional relationships among individuals, by name, who are treating him.

9. The patient has the right to be advised if the hospital proposes to engage in or perform human experimentation affecting his care or treatment. The patient has the right to refuse to participate in such research projects.

10. The patient has the right to expect reasonable continuity of care. He has the right to know in advance what appointment times and physicians are available and where. The patient has the right to expect that the hospital will provide a mechanism whereby he is informed by his physician or a delegate of the physician of the patient's continuing health care requirements following discharge.

11. The patient has the right to examine and receive an explanation of his bill regardless of source of payment.

12. The patient has the right to know what hospital rules and regulations apply to his conduct as a patient.

No catalog of rights can guarantee for the patient the kind of treatment he has a right to expect. A hospital has many functions to perform, including the prevention and treatment of disease, the education of both health professionals and patients, and the conduct of clinical research. All these activities must be conducted with an overriding concern for the patient, and, above all, the recognition of his dignity as a human being. Success in achieving this recognition assures success in the defense of the rights of the patient.

(Approved by the American Hospital Association House of Delegates, February 6, 1973, and reprinted by permission of the American Hospital Association.)

- Consider this Bill of Rights, as a possible patient, and as a professional. Do these roles conflict when you read this Bill?

In Britain the introduction of the Citizens' Charter and the associated Patients' Charter and Primary Care Charter set out a similar series of rights for patients and the public. The following is the Patients' Charter, in the Scottish version.

The NHS in Scotland exists to serve the community

by promoting good health
by treating those who are ill, and
by providing continuing health care to those who need it.

Improving health in Scotland

You are entitled
to have a say about how to improve health locally
to information and help to keep as healthy as possible
You should share in the responsibility for your own health.

Improving care for patients

You are entitled
to the highest standards possible for yourself, your family and your friends
to be treated as a person, not a case
to understandable explanations
to access (with safeguards) to information held about you, and to

be sure that this information will be kept confidential
to be involved so far as is practical in making decisions about
your health and wherever possible to be given choices
to expect close links between different people providing your care
to expect that all NHS staff will ask themselves 'How would I want
to be treated if it were me?'.

Reduced waiting times

You are entitled
to be treated as quickly as possible
as from April 1992 to a guarantee of admission to
hospital within a set period, with special priority for
those waiting in pain and discomfort
to know how long you are likely to wait in the
waiting room
**You should help us to help you by turning up
on time and letting us know if you have to
cancel or have changed your address.**

Tell us what you think

**We want to know what you think, good or bad,
about the care you have received. This will
help identify how we can—and will—do better
in future.**

You are entitled
to have your comments or complaints treated fairly
and quickly
to help and advice eg from your local health council
to a clear and courteous answer.

Improving information

To help you, the NHS in Scotland is to provide
more information about health services and the NHS.

What has been done already

GPs and Dentists have agreed
- to put more emphasis on health promotion and preventing
  illness

- to offer a more responsive service with more choice, more information
- to offer consultations to new patients, patients not seen for 3 years and annual consultation to those aged 75 and over.

Health Education Board for Scotland has been set up to lead health education drive at national level.

Targets have been set for improving health in Scotland by the year 2000.

Great progress has been made in setting standards for health care, and introducing clinical audit to review these standards.

Three quarters of all NHS patients are treated within 4 weeks.

Target times have been set for key specialties within which 9 out of 10 people must be treated.

Raising the Standard

Health Boards will shortly announce further plans and initiatives to improve the health of their local population.

Higher standards of care will be developed and published in patient's charters in all hospitals, community and other health services.

Health Boards will *guarantee* to treat patients within a set time in certain key specialties.

For the very small number of people who presently wait for a long time for treatment, there will be a *national* guarantee of treatment within 18 months. This will be subject to certain very limited exceptions (such as availability of organs for transplants).

Targets for waiting times for outpatient appointments will be set and published.

This leaflet is a summary of the proposals contained in The Scottish Office Patient's Charter published in September 1991 which is available from Health Boards and local Health Councils.

- What are the advantages and disadvantages of having such charters?

6. DECLARATION OF HELSINKI

The World Medical Association have drawn up a code of practice in relation to Biomedical Research. All concerned in research should be aware of this, as, of all the codes discussed, it is the most specific. It first reviews general principles, then the problems of clinical research. Finally, it covers the important topic of volunteers in research.

The World Medical Association Declaration of Helsinki

Introduction

It is the mission of the medical doctor to safeguard the health of the people. His or her knowledge and conscience are dedicated to the fulfilment of this mission.

The Declaration of Geneva of the World Medical Association binds the doctor with the words, 'The health of my patient will be my first consideration', and the International Code of Medical Ethics declares that, 'Any act or advice which could weaken physical or mental resistance of a human being may be used only in his interest.'

The purpose of biomedical research involving human subjects must be to improve diagnostic, therapeutic and prophylactic procedures and the understanding of the aetiology and pathogenesis of disease.

In current medical practice most diagnostic, therapeutic or prophylactic procedures involve hazards. This applies *a fortiori* in biomedical research. Medical progress is based on research which ultimately must rest in part on experimentation involving human subjects.

In the field of biomedical research a fundamental distinction must be recognized between medical research in which the aim is essentially diagnostic or therapeutic for a patient, and medical research, the essential object of which is purely scientific and without direct diagnostic or therapeutic value to the person subjected to the research.

Special caution must be exercised in the conduct of research which may affect the environment, and the welfare of animals used for research must be respected.

Because it is essential that the results of laboratory experiments be applied to human beings to further scientific knowledge and to help suffering humanity, the World Medical Association has prepared the following recommendations as a guide to every doctor in biomedical research involving human subjects. They should be kept under review in the future. It must be stressed that the standards as drafted are only a guide to physicians all over the world. Doctors are not relieved from criminal, civil and ethical responsibilities under the laws of their own countries.

I. Basic principles

1. Biomedical research involving human subjects must conform to generally accepted scientific principles and should be based on adequately performed laboratory and animal experimentation and on a thorough knowledge of the scientific literature.

2. The design and performance of each experimental procedure involving human subjects should be clearly formulated in an experimental protocol which should be transmitted to a specially appointed independent committee for consideration, comment and guidance.

3. Biomedical research involving human subjects should be conducted only by scientifically qualified persons and under the supervision of a clinically competent medical person. The responsibility for the human subject must always rest with a medically qualified person and never rest on the subject of the research, even though the subject has given his or her consent.

4. Biomedical research involving human subjects cannot legitimately be carried out unless the importance of the objective is in proportion to the inherent risk to the subject.

5. Every biomedical research project involving human subjects should be preceded by careful assessment of predictable risks in comparison with foreseeable benefits to the subject or to others. Concern for the interests of the subject must always prevail over the interests of science and society.

6. The right of the research subject to safeguard his or her integrity must always be respected. Every precaution should be taken to respect the privacy of the subject and to minimize the impact of the study on the subject's physical and mental integrity and on the personality of the subject.

7. Doctors should abstain from engaging in research projects involving human subjects unless they are satisfied that the hazards involved are believed to be predictable. Doctors should cease any investigation if the hazards are found to outweigh the potential benefits.

8. In publication of the results of his or her research, the doctor is obliged to preserve the accuracy of the results. Reports of experimentation not in accordance with the principles laid down in this Declaration should not be accepted for publication.

9. In any research on human beings, each potential subject must be adequately informed of the aims, methods, anticipated benefits and potential hazards of the study and the discomfort it may entail. He or she should be informed that he or she is at liberty to abstain from participation in the study and that he or she is free to withdraw his or her consent to participation at any time. The doctor should then obtain the subject's freely-given informed consent, preferably in writing.

10. When obtaining informed consent for the research project the doctor should be particularly cautious if the subject is in a dependent relationship to him or her or may consent under duress. In that case the informed consent should be obtained by a doctor who is not engaged in the investigation and who is completely independent of this official relationship.

11. In the case of legal incompetence, informed consent should be obtained from the legal guardian in accordance with national legislation. Where physical or mental incapacity makes it impossible to obtain informed consent, or when the subject is a minor, permission from the responsible relative replaces that of the subject in accordance with national legislation.

12. The research protocol should always contain a statement of the ethical consideration involved and should indicate that the principles enunciated in the present Declaration are complied with.

II. Medical research combined with professional care (clinical research)

1. In the treatment of the sick person, the doctor must be free to use a new diagnostic and therapeutic measure, if in his or her judgement it offers hope of saving life, re-establishing health or alleviating suffering.

2. The potential benefits, hazards and discomfort of a new method should be weighed against the advantages of the best current diagnostic and therapeutic methods.

3. In any medical study, every patient—including those of a control group, if any—should be assured of the best proven diagnostic and therapeutic method.

4. The refusal of the patient to participate in a study must never interfere with the doctor-patient relationship.

5. If the doctor considers it essential not to obtain informed consent, the specific reasons for this proposal should be stated in the experimental protocol for transmission to the independent committee (1, 2).

6. The doctor can combine medical research with professional care, the objective being the acquisition of new medical knowledge, only to the extent that medical research is justified by its potential diagnostic or therapeutic value for the patient.

III. Non-therapeutic biomedical research involving human subjects (non-clinical biomedical research)

1. In the purely scientific application of medical research carried out on a human being, it is the duty of the doctor to remain the protector of the life and health of that person on whom biomedical research is being carried out.

2. The subjects should be volunteers—either healthy persons or patients for whom the experimental design is not related to the patient's illness.

3. The investigator or the investigating team should discontinue the research if in his/her or their judgment it may, if continued, be harmful to the individual.

4. In research on man, the interest of science and society should never take precedence over considerations related to the wellbeing of the subject.

(Adopted by the 18th World Medical Assembly, Helsinki, Finland, 1964, and as revised by the 29th World Medical Assembly, Tokyo, Japan, 1975. Reprinted by permission.)

● Consider this declaration and decide whether or not you can agree with all of its guide-lines? Does II.3 contradict itself?

7. CONCLUSION

We have listed here only a sample of the many codes of ethics available. They are more or less specific and, though there is overlap, there are real variations in the content of such codes.

● Having read them, how valuable do you now think they are?
● If you were invited to join a panel of members of your own professional group to draw up a 'new' code of ethics, would you agree to take part? What would be the content of 'your' code?

BIBLIOGRAPHY

1. Classical sources

The classical sources of the philosophy we have put forward can be found in the following works which are published in many editions:

Plato, *Republic, Meno, Protagoras*
Aristotle, *Nicomachean ethics*
Hume, D. *Treatise of human nature*, Book III
Kant, I. *Groundwork of the metaphysic of morals*
Mill, J.S. *Utilitarianism* and *On Liberty*

2. Moral philosophy

The following are a few of the many approachable books on moral philosophy:

Benn, S.I. and Peters, R.S. (1971). *Social principles and the democratic state*, 2nd edn. George Allen & Unwin, London.
Campbell, T. (1988). *Justice*. Macmillan, London.
Downie, R.S. (1977). *Roles and values* (3rd impression). Methuen, London.
MacIntyre, A. (1967). *A short history of ethics*. Routledge & Kegan Paul, London. (Also Macmillan paperback, New York.)
Mackie, J.L. (1977). *Ethics*. Pelican, Harmondsworth.
Midgley, M. (1977). *Heart and mind*. Methuen, London.
Rachels, J. (1986). *The elements of moral philosophy*. Random House, New York.
Raphael, D.D. (1981). *Moral philosophy*. Oxford University Press, Oxford.
Singer, P. (1979). *Practical ethics*. Cambridge University Press, Cambridge.
Stevenson, L. (1974). *Seven theories of human nature*. Oxford University Press, Oxford.
Torrance, G.W. (1986). *Journal of Health Economics*, **5**, 1–30.

3. Health care ethics

Beauchamp, T.L. and Childress, J.F. (1983). *Principles of biomedical ethics*, 2nd edn. Oxford University Press, New York.

Benjamin, M. and Curtis, J. (1988). *Ethics in nursing*. Oxford University Press, New York.

Boyd, K.M., Melia, K.M., and Thomson, I.E. (1983). *Nursing ethics*. Churchill Livingstone, Edinburgh.

Brody, B. (1988). *Life and death decision making*. Oxford University Press, Oxford.

Campbell, A.V. (1984). *Moral dilemmas in medicine*, 3rd edn. Churchill Livingstone, Edinburgh.

Central Council for Education and Training in Social Work (CCETSW). (1976). *Values in social work*, CCETSW Paper 13. CCETSW, London.

Culver, C. and Gert, B. (1982). *Philosophy in medicine*. Oxford University Press, New York.

Downie, R.S. and Charlton, B. (1992). *The making of a doctor*. Oxford University Press, Oxford.

Glover, J. (1977). *Causing death and saving lives*. Penguin, Harmondsworth.

Harris, J. (1985). *The value of life*. Routledge & Kegan Paul, London.

Illich, I. (1978). *Limits to medicine (medical nemesis)*. Penguin, Harmondsworth.

Jennett, B. (1984). *High technology medicine*. Nuffield Provincial Hospitals Trust, London.

Kennedy, Ian. (1983). *The unmasking of medicine*. Paladin, London.

Gillon, R. (1987). *Philosophical medical ethics*. Wiley, Chichester.

Gilligan, C. (1982). *In a different voice*. Harvard University Press, Boston.

Gallagher, U. and Boyd, K. (1991). *Teaching and learning nursing ethics*. Scutari Press, London.

Gorovitz, S. (1991). *Drawing the line*. Oxford University Press, New York.

Lockwood, M. (ed.) (1985). *Moral dilemmas in modern medicine*. Oxford University Press, New York.

McCloskey, J.C. and Grace, H.K. (1981). *Current issues in nursing*. Blackwell Scientific Publications, Oxford.

McLean, S.A.M. (ed.) (1981). *Legal issues in medicine*. Gower, Aldershot.

Melia, K.M. (1987). *Everyday nursing ethics*. Macmillan, London.

Muyskens, J.L. (1982). *Moral problems in nursing*. Rowman & Littlefield, Totowa, New Jersey.

Pellegrino, E.D. and Thomasma, D.C. (1981). *A philosophical basis of medical practice*. Oxford University Press, New York.

Pence, G. (1980). *Ethical options in medicine*. Medical Economics Books, Oradell, New Jersey.

Plant, R. (1970). *Social and moral theory in casework*. Routledge & Kegan Paul, London.

Rumbold, G. (1986).*Ethics in nursing practice*. Ballière Tindall, London.

Warnock, M. (1985). *A question of life*. Basil Blackwell, Oxford.

Zorza, R. and Zorza, V. (1980). *A way to die*. Sphere Books, London.

4. Collections of essays

Ladd, J. (1979). *Ethical issues relating to life and death*. Oxford University Press, New York.

Rachels, J. (1975). *Moral problems*. Harper & Row, New York.

Steinbock, B. (1980). *Killing and letting die*. Prentice-Hall, Englewood Cliffs, New Jersey.

Walters, W. and Singer, P. (1982). *Test tube babies*. Oxford University Press, Melbourne.

5. Reference books

In researching a specific topic the reader may first consult the brief entries (with references) in the following:

Duncan, A.A., Dunstan, G.R., and Welbourn, R.B. (1981). *Dictionary of medical ethics*, 2nd edn. Darton, Longman & Todd, London.

For more detailed treatment and fuller references the following resources are also available:

Reich, W.T. (1978). *Encyclopaedia of bioethics*, 4 volumes. Macmillan and Free Press, New York and London.

Walters, L. (Published annually) *Bibliography of bioethics*. Macmillan and Free Press, New York and London.

6. Journals

Journal of Medical Ethics
Journal of Medicine and Philosophy
Journal of Applied Philosophy
Bioethics.

7. Logic and the philosophy of science

Chalmers, A.F. (1978). *What is this thing called science?* The Open University, Milton Keynes.

Flew, A. (1985). *Thinking about thinking*. Fontana, London.

Salmon, W. (1973). *Logic*, 2nd edn. Prentice-Hall, Englewood Cliffs, New Jersey.

Shaw, P. (1981). *Logic and its limits*. Pan Books, London and Sydney.

8. Literature and moral education

(a) General works about the use of literature in health care education.

Billings, J.A., Coles, R., Reiser, S.J., and Stoeckle, J.D. (1985). A seminar in 'plain doctoring'. *Journal of Medical Education*, 60, November.

Brody, H. (1987). *Stories of sickness*. Yale University Press, New Haven and London.

Callahan, D., Caplan, A., and Jennings, B. (1984). *On the uses of the humanities*. The Hastings Center, New York.

Cassell, E.J. (1984). *The place of the humanities in medicine*. The Hastings Center, New York.

Millard, D.A. (1977). Literature and the therapeutic imagination. *British Journal of Social Work*, **7**, 2.

(b) A few suggested literary sources:

Downie, R.S. (1994). *The healing arts: an Oxford anthology*. Oxford University Press, Oxford/New York.

Enright, D.J. (1989). *The Faber book of fevers and frets*. Faber, London.

Lowbury, E. (1990). *Apollo*. Keynes Press, London.

Porter, R. (1991). *The Faber book of madness*. Faber, London.

INDEX